GREENER PASTURES CALLING

ONCE UPON A VET SCHOOL: PRACTICE TIME

LIZZI TREMAYNE

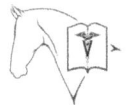

New Zealand and United States Copyright 2018 by Lizzi Tremayne

All rights reserved. No part of this publication may be reproduced, distributed or transmitted in any form or by any means, without prior written permission.

Lizzi Tremayne / Blue Mist Publishing

Franklin Road, RD 2

Waihi, New Zealand 3682

www.lizzitremayne.com

Publisher's Note: This is a work of fiction. Names, characters, places, and incidents are a product of the author's imagination. Locales and public names are sometimes used for atmospheric purposes. Any resemblance to actual people, living or dead, or to businesses, companies, events, institutions, or locales is completely coincidental.

Formatting, cover design, photos, and artwork by Lizzi Tremayne

Cover photo credit to Kirsten Petersen and Lizzi Tremayne

Author photo credit to Kajai@gmail.com

Previously published with Authors of Main Street in Anthology: Christmas Wishes on Main Street 4 November 2018

From the **Practice Time** sequence of the **Once Upon a Vet School** series

Greener Pastures Calling / Lizzi Tremayne 1st Edition December 2018

Printed in New Zealand and the United States of America

Paperback Edition 2019 08 29-V6

ISBN 978-0-9951157-1-2

DEDICATED TO

Dedicated to

John and Janet Harrison

John:

Thank you for taking a risk on the first girl horse vet in your practice—a *Yank*, no less—so very long ago and taking me under your wing. You taught me cows are so much more than a black and white box I couldn't previously see inside. And all about road user charges—sorry to take ten years off your life.

Your 'nonexistent' (read: *hidden*) skills in small animal surgery which I was blessed to see (read: *caught you at*) that day in the clinic astounded me. I figure by now it's safe to 'let the cat out of the bag' that this cow vet is a brilliant small animal surgeon. To this day, I've never seen such delicate tissue handling.

That little cat probably never even knew she'd been spayed.

Janet:

Thank you for welcoming me into your home and your family when John took this waif from California into the practice, shocking as I might have been. Your dry humor warmed me on many otherwise very chilly days.

The twins (who have children of their own by now) were gorgeous and your beautiful daughter, sharp girl that she was even at eleven, taught me more about global affairs than I'd learned in the States in my entire lifetime.

It certainly explained why so many Kiwis thought Yanks didn't give a hoot about other countries. Unless they had highly educated parents and watched BBC or such, they were only presented with domestic affairs… and they didn't *know* about the rest of the world.

Thank you both for making a huge difference to my life.

CONTENTS

Books by Lizzi Tremayne   vii
Praise for Lizzi Tremayne   ix
Glossary of Kiwi and Other Terms   xvii

Chapter 1	1
Chapter 2	11
Chapter 3	21
Chapter 4	33
Chapter 5	43
Chapter 6	53
Chapter 7	61
Chapter 8	69
Chapter 9	79
Chapter 10	85
Chapter 11	95
Chapter 12	101
Epilogue	105
Find Books	109
Books by the Author	111
Author's Notes	121
Recipe: Whitebait Fritters	123
About the Author	125
Connect with Lizzi	127
Acknowledgements	129
Excerpt from A Long Trail Rolling	131
Excerpt from Tatiana	141

BOOKS BY LIZZI TREMAYNE

The Long Trails Series
A Long Trail Rolling (Book One)
The Hills of Gold Unchanging (Book Two)
A Sea of Green Unfolding (Book Three)

Multi-Series Samplers
Lizzi Tremayne First Chapter Sampler

The *Once Upon a Vet School* Series
~Vet School 24/7~
Fifty Miles at a Breath
Lena Takes a Foal
~Practice Time~
Greener Pastures Calling

Boxed sets with Authors of Main Street
Christmas Babies on Main Street
Summer Romance on Main Street
Christmas Wishes on Main Street

Boxed sets with Bluestocking Belles
Follow Your Star Home

Sign up for Lizzi's VIP Readers Club to hear about new releases and specials, plus get your free sampler gift here:

www.lizzitremayne.com/VIPGreen

PRAISE FOR LIZZI TREMAYNE

With her debut novel, A Long Trail Rolling, *Lizzi was:*

Winner 2016 True West Magazine
Best Western Romance
Winner 2015 RWNZ Koru Award
Finalist 2015 Best Indie Book Award
Winner 2014 RWNZ Pacific Hearts Award
Finalist 2013 RWNZ Great Beginnings

"vivid, light and fast-paced… a ripping good read."
 –*Deborah Challinor, number one bestselling author and historian*

"An authentic, emotional story of one woman's fight for survival in an unforgiving landscape."

–Leeanna Morgan, USA Today bestselling author

"An impressive debut…a romance, a western, and an adventure story, all rolled up into a compelling read."
–Booksellers NZ

The Hills of Gold Unchanging:
"The pace is fast, there's plenty of action and adventure and a few twists I didn't see coming. Good characters plus excellent history equals a great read."
–Deborah Challinor, number one bestselling author and historian

"…superb storytelling."
–Judy Knighton, editor

"I particularly liked the attention to historical detail. This is an author who does her homework, and it shows… a cracking good yarn."
–Shelagh Merlin, NetGalley Reviewer

A Sea of Green Unfolding:
"the historical research is excellent…well-integrated into the narrative."
–Deborah Challinor, number one bestselling author and historian

"A lovely combination of historical accuracy and adventure…[a] beautifully researched and engrossing story."

—*Shelagh Merlin, NetGalley reviewer*

"Loved this book. The characters draw you in on a story filled with interest and suspense."
—*Kate Le Petit*

Fifty Miles at a Breath

"Lizzi Tremayne is a born storyteller. The…characters… [are] three dimensional and you can feel Lena and Blake's emotions."
—*Lori Dykes*

"a wonderful series about the path to becoming a veterinarian, the love of horses and sweet romance. Lena and Blake will grab your heart."
—*Teri Donaldson*

Lena Takes a Foal

"This book is for anyone with a passion for horses… or anyone who loves a story about strong, independent young women finding love!"
—*Stacey*

"The story… displays Lizzi Tremayne's ability to develop strong characters… with a nice strong black moment to challenge our heroine and prove her worth."
—*Shelagh Merlin, NetGalley Reviewer*

"...the perfect blend of sweet romance, horses and real emotions with fascinating information woven in about the medical care of horses."
 —*Teri Donaldson*

"As I turned the last page I cannot stop smiling! I look forward to more in this series and from this author!!!"
 —*Lori Dykes*

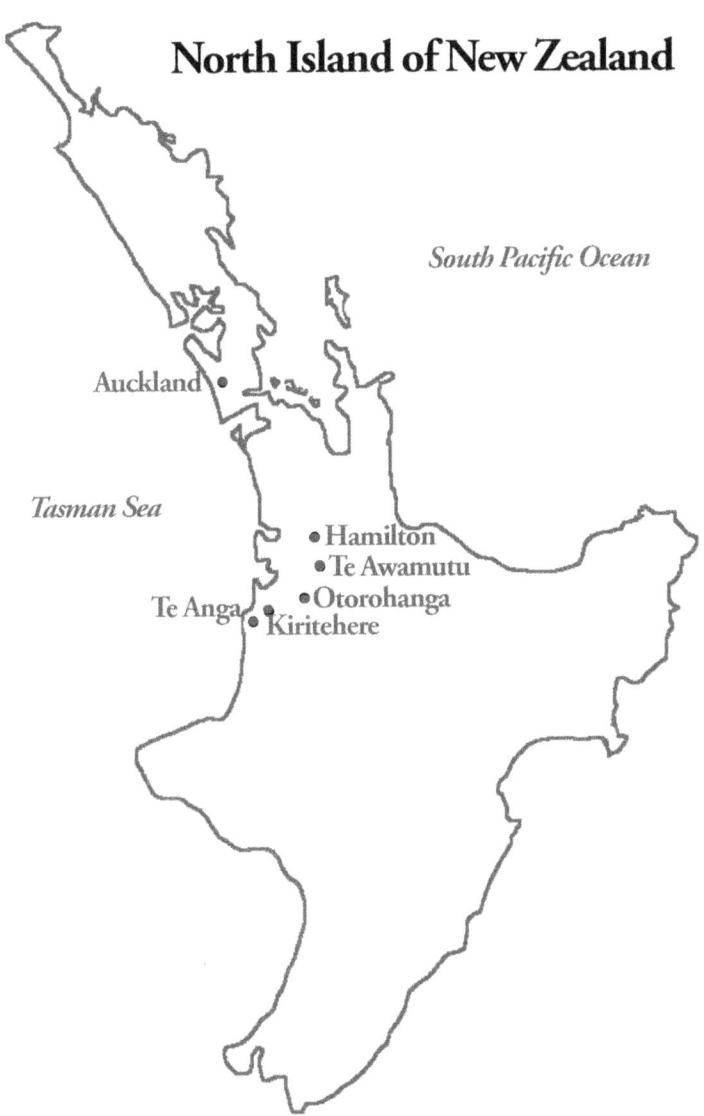

Hamilton to Kiritehere

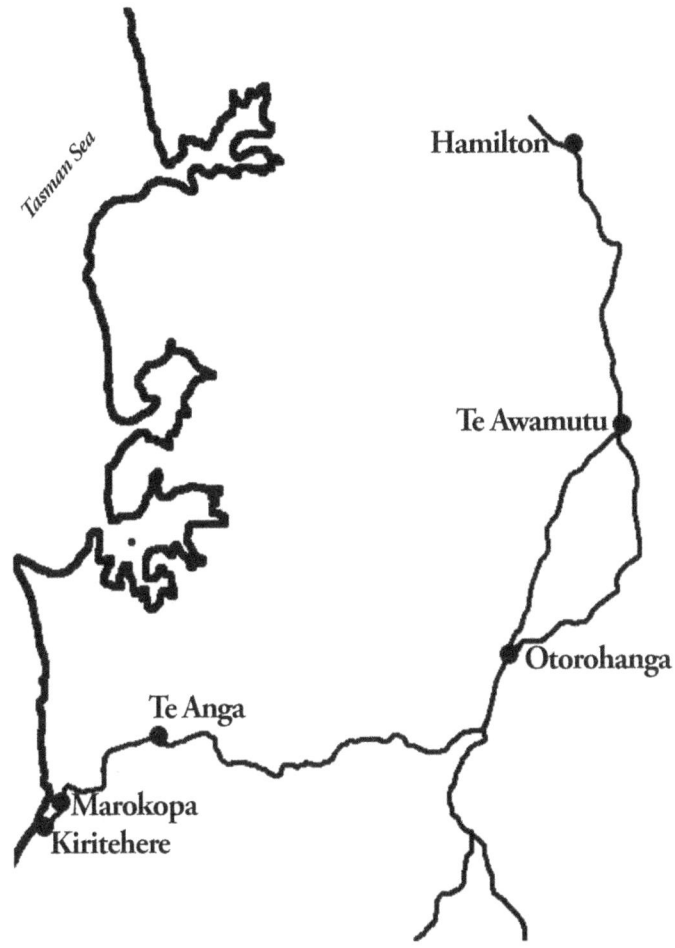

GLOSSARY OF KIWI AND OTHER TERMS

a little off ~ mildly lame

bach ~ summer beach house

bikkies ~ cookies, short for biscuits

biro ~ ball point pen

block ~ piece of land, anything from a small section to a farm

butter safe ~ historically, a cabinet built into a kitchen with netting to the outside to keep food cool, especially eggs and dairy

chocker ~ full

deal to ~ to sort out | e.g., to "deal to him" is to sort him out, probably physically

down the line ~ heading south | The old North-South railway "line" running through the country was the only way to get anywhere in days past

dummy ~ pacifier for a baby | e.g., to "spit the dummy" is to have hysterics, like a baby spitting out their dummy | cf. "to pack/ chuck a wobbly"

esky ~ ice cooler or chilly bin

Fresian ~ what Kiwis call Holstein-Fresian cows | also a horse breed, but not for this book

good on ya ~ well done

ice cream container ~ the Kiwi equivalent of US coffee cans | e.g. "I feed him 2 ice cream containers of chaff and one of sweet feed, Doc."

metal ~ gravel, small rocks

newbie ~ newcomer to anything like a sport or hobby

rang off/ring off ~ the act of hanging up the phone

staring ~ dull haircoat with no gloss, hair standing on end

stock agent ~ stock buyer and seller, one who organizes for a cow to be "put on the truck" with destination slaughterhouse or sale | Akin to used car salesmen

stunned mullet ~ the look of a fish which has been stunned: open mouth and staring eyes, stupefied

tar-seal ~ road surface made by pouring hot tar on base layer and spreading metal over the top | cf. **metal**, above

three-legged lame ~ an animal so lame it can't bear weight on one of its four legs

togs ~ bathing suit

track ~ trail or dirt road

tucker ~ feed | e.g.: "off his tucker", or not eating

ute ~ "utility vehicle", or mini pickup truck

wobbly ~ tantrum or fit, hysterics e.g., to "chuck" or "pack" a wobbly" is to throw a tantrum—think of a 2 1/2 year old who wants a toy. Badly. They wobble, don't they? | cf. **dummy**, above

1

September 1992, Te Awamutu, New Zealand

AFTER ONE LOOK inside the cowshed at 25 Wharewhero Road, I didn't think I'd ever be able to touch even my favorite Tip Top Chocolate Ice Cream again… not ever.

And that was before the putrid odor hit me.

"Eh, where's the vet?" someone called from the pit between the cows and I peered down into the darkness. Sure enough, there was a little man in there, barely visible. His overalls were so crusted with unmentionables that he was hard to distinguish from the oily, black muck covering every surface of the shed—rails, floor, and halfway up the walls.

I swallowed hard and forced my gorge to stay down.

"I'm here," I called from the doorway. I wanted to leave and never come back, but after glancing at the miserable-looking cows standing in the row, I picked my way through the morass covering the floor and stepped down into the pit. I froze a meter away from the man, my eyes watering. He smelled, if possible, worse than his shed.

My God, didn't the dairy factory monitor these places?

As he hadn't said anything more, I gazed past him to the far end of the shed where the six cows stood with their heads down, eyes lackluster, and coats staring. From each of the cows' backsides hung the rotting remnants of their calf fetal membranes. I guess something *could* smell worse than this man.

"So why'd they send a girl?" The man's brows narrowed over a pursed mouth.

"They sent a veterinarian. I'm Dr. Scott. Nice to meet you… Mr. Somerfield, I presume?" I said, dryly, then turned to the cows.

He nodded once in reply.

"How long ago did these girls calve?"

"Ah," his scowl remained undiminished, but he seemed at a loss, "some a week, some more, maybe two weeks."

I scanned the row of dejected, probably septic, cows and held back a shudder of revulsion. "That long?" I gritted my teeth to keep from screaming at him.

"I didn't want to waste my money, what with having the vets come out too many times."

"It costs less to—" I stopped and shut my trap before it got me into trouble again and spun back toward the ute. "Please put them into the vet race so I can treat them properly," I called over my shoulder, not trusting myself to say more. I rather liked my job with the practice.

Tossing gloves, disinfectant, antibiotics, needles and

syringes, a fluid pump, and an old stomach tube into several buckets, I prepared for the ordeal ahead. By the clanging of pipe gates and shouting behind me, at least I knew he was moving the cows.

When I returned to the shed, Somerfield's eyes bugged at the buckets weighing me down. I could see him ticking off the fees in his head. "You don't need all that, just some foaming pessaries and you'll be away."

I locked my jaw as I stared at him. Setting down the buckets, I pulled a thermometer from my pocket. With a deep breath, I tried for patience while I lubed the thing and inserted it gently into the first cow's rectum. "Mr. Somerfield," I finally said, "if you'd rung a week or two ago, that might have been all we needed. As it is," I removed the thermometer and glanced at it, shook it down, and replaced it to double-check the ridiculously high temperature, "it appears these cows are far past simple antibiotic pessaries."

He jerked his head toward me for a moment then scowled. "They're just soft," he muttered, and stalked away. The cows, to a one, cringed away as he passed them. Never a good sign.

I consulted the thermometer again. *41 degrees C...* over 105 degrees F. I let my breath out and checked the next cow. Her temperature wasn't far below that, nor the next.

When he came back, I turned to him, my face as impassive as I could make it. "Mr. Somerfield, your cows are septic. They have very bad infections. I'm going to try to remove what's left of their placentas, flush out their uteri, and put antibiotics in, plus give them intravenous antibiotics. I'll return tomorrow. I'll not lie to you, you may lose some of them. They are *that* sick."

By the look on his face—the stunned mullet look, as they call it in New Zealand—I could see he finally understood the gravity of the situation.

I was finally all dressed up for the party in my calving gown and doubled rectal sleeves, with exam gloves over the top. A bit pathetic, of course; they all leaked within minutes.

I cleaned the first cow's backside as best I could with a running hose and disinfectant before lubing up and starting. With the time that'd elapsed since she calved, it was a struggle to get my hand through the mostly-closed cervix of that first cow. My goal was to somehow remove whatever tissues hadn't yet liquified, then to flush whatever remained. Tricky business.

There's nothing quite like the scent of two-week-old rotting tissue, but as always, I employed the standard tactic learned by every veterinary student in formalin-filled labs: I blocked my nose to the smells and breathed through my mouth.

While a calving or a prolapsed uterus on a cow probably took more sheer strength, "cleaning" a cow of its retained fetal membranes was probably the most truly unpleasant job I knew. For both the vet *and* the cow. And this farm didn't have the usual one or two, but six.

It took hours.

Needless to say, by the end of it, I was covered. Wisps of my long hair, once clipped back and braided to within an inch of their lives, had escaped their fetters and now straggled down around my face. And I'm sure I smeared the back of my none-too-clean gloves across my cheek more than once.

I couldn't wait to get back to the clinic for a much-needed shower.

Even Somerville bordered on chartreuse beneath his grime by the time we were done. He, of course, got the job of holding the cows' tails and pumping fluid through the tube when I needed it. He was drowned by the upset cows' excrement more than once. I'm sure I didn't fully escape it, either, but at least it wasn't on my head.

"I'll see you tomorrow," I said lightly to Mr. Somerville, after the last cow had been injected with antibiotics and he'd opened the gate to let her out.

He only nodded and kept his head down.

Heaving a great sigh, I picked up my grotty buckets and headed for the vat room to give my gear a perfunctory wash —nothing was going into my vehicle in its current state, including me. A few moments later, as it steamed into my buckets, the water from the ever-present, blessed boiler looked almost warm enough to do the job.

I picked up a scrubbing brush from beside the tank, then dropped it back to the floor—I'd get my own. This one was as disgusting as everything else on the place.

Still too filthy to even touch my door handles, I ducked down to rinse my hands and arms from the cold hose.

Somewhere out on the tanker track loop, a vehicle door slammed.

"Somerfield?" A loud male voice rang out only moments later in the doorway beside me.

I glanced up to see a young man stride in. His face red and angry, he stared through the open doors of the vat room toward the cowshed from his considerable height and nearly tripped over me. He looked down in horror and our eyes locked as he stopped in his tracks. I'd like to think it was my beauty, but I suspect it was mostly the smell.

"I wouldn't get too close if I were you," I said faintly, unable to look away. "You might smell like this forever."

"Oh, I'm sorry," he said. He glanced away, then back, and offered me a strained smile. "I was looking for Somerfield."

"I gathered that." I raised a brow at him, wishing I didn't look like a veterinary ghoul. "He's in there. Looking rather green, I might add." I flicked my head back toward the shed and some bedraggled tendrils of what used to be hair slapped against my face. I shuddered and closed my eyes, wishing I were anywhere else.

"You okay there?" His voice, when it wasn't at full noise, was smooth as old port.

"I will be after I'm gone"— I gulped and tried not to look into his extraordinary eyes again—"and I've soaked in a bubble bath for a week."

"I'll leave you to it, then." A grin cracked his visage as he passed me. "Good luck."

He didn't return before I managed to scrub the worst off my gear and roll it up inside my calving gown. I shoved the packet into one of the buckets and glanced over my shoulder to see the man gesticulating wildly at the cringing Somerfield.

Good on him. Somebody needed to do that.

As I drove around the roundabout heading for the gate, he stepped out the door and waved.

Just my luck the only guy I'd met in New Zealand who looked like he could've graced the covers of GQ had to meet me when I looked as if I'd just been dragged through a cesspool.

"Come on, Lena, it'll be fun," Moira said, reaching high above her head to shove the last box of dry-cow mastitis therapy into its place. "You haven't gone out with a guy since you went rock-and-rolling with that wet noodle in Hamilton. That was ages ago."

I winced. My toes still hurt, even three months later. "He talked a good line. I thought he could dance."

"Yeah, well, you should've listened to me, but you were so desperate to hit a dance floor, you went anyway."

"What can I say? I've missed dancing terribly since I left the States—that and missing out on the veterinary acupuncture course I'd booked before I left."

"The one you've nearly completed now in Australia?" she said, with a twist of her lips.

I laughed at her. "Okay, so things are looking up. Now it's just the dancing I miss."

"That, and a good Kiwi Bloke to go along with it."

"Mmm…" I'd picked up the wonderful Kiwi term that can mean anything from agreement to disagreement, from *absolutely!* to f-off—and only the speaker knows what he or she meant. Handy. We don't have anything like it in America.

Granted, I was generally either working or sleeping these days, but the Kiwi men I'd met so far seemed to be either married farmers or usually-drunk rugby boys—neither of which appealed.

"I've got an idea. I know this guy—"

"Been there, Moira, not going there again. Your blind dates… lack… *something*. I daren't elaborate. I'm meant to have a clean mouth here." I looked around the front showroom of the big veterinary clinic.

The equine section of the display floor was currently limited to a one by two-meter area of shelf space. The rest of the massive showroom was dedicated to cattle—specifically, dairy cattle—medicines and supplements, but I was working on that. I'd been hired to service the equine side of the practice, taking over from a man who'd been the sole equine practitioner in this area for the past thirty-three years. It would take some doing to convince some of the racing guys that the first female vet this practice had ever hired—and one the age of their granddaughters to boot—was worth her salt.

"Lena?"

I blinked. Moira looked at me, one brow raised. "Yes?" I mumbled.

"Really?" Her eyes widened and her mouth dropped open.

"Pardon?"

She laughed. You said yes to double dating with Mark and me."

"Sorry"—I frowned—"I didn't hear you."

"It'll be fun. He's nice. You'll like him."

"Who?"

"Marcus. He's a stock agent—with a gorgeous Holden."

"Stock agent." I close my eyes and took a deep breath.

"They're okay," she assured me, with a laugh.

"Bit like a used car salesman, if you ask me."

"Well… maybe, but it'll be fun."

I shook my head and rubbed my forehead. "So, what have you cooked up?"

"Fawlty Towers dinner and show."

"Where? I haven't seen it advertised."

"Well," she squirmed a little, "it's down the line a little ways."

"I see." I stared her down. "Like how far down the line?"

"Ummm…"—she hesitated, then went on quickly"—"Taumarunui, but it'll be fun."

"Taumarunui? That's hours away." I dragged in another deep breath. "Okay, I'll go, but we'll drive together, right?"

"Of course. It's on Saturday night."

I didn't like the thought of the nearly two hours of questionable roads"—each way. That show had better be good.

2

The show *was* good, hysterical even, but my date, Marcus, got progressively more drunk as the evening went on. Obnoxiously drunk, to boot. I was trying to figure out how to get the keys for his shiny black Holden out of his hand and into mine, because as luck would have it, Moira had to cancel to care for her injured sister's children. How could I complain about that?

So here I was, wondering at my brilliance for getting into this situation, feeling trapped, and wondering what to do next. The concept of a bus way out here was a joke—and a taxi? I didn't make enough money for that, if a taxi stand even existed in this little backwater town.

"Arm-wrestle for the key?" Marcus laughed playfully.

Asking nicely for the keychain hadn't worked. It seems Marcus thought it all a bit of fun.

Drinking and driving just wasn't done, where I'd come from. Unfortunately, it was treated lightly here. New Zealand's rugby culture, with its associated "drinkies" in the clubroom before going—*driving*—home, was strong. It wasn't confined to the rugby boys, though. The culture spread across many sports—and it didn't bear thinking about.

And it appeared I was about to go home with *this* drunk. Not bloody likely, if I had anything to say about it.

"Arm-wrestle *you*, you big galumph?" I finally answered, trying to keep the knife edge from my voice. I don't think I succeeded, but he didn't seem to notice.

I gave it my best, but then, rubbing my sore arm, I tried cajoling, also to no avail.

By this time, only the servers remained.

"No, none of us live up north," whispered one.

"*Very sorry*," another said, wincing as she took in the condition of my erstwhile "date".

In the end, I trusted to Providence, but still cursed Moira, him, myself, and anyone else I could think of.

An hour on, as we drove through Otorohranga, Marcus turned due north toward Te Awamutu on the narrow backroad which wound on past Te Kawa and toward Pokuru. I tried not to stare out into the dark, tried to forget about the ditches and sheer banks I knew dropped away just past the sides of the road.

Marcus nattered on as we drove north. From the sideways glances he kept sending in my direction, I suspected he might be sobering up. "I'm so tired" he said, as we clattered over a railway bridge. "What say we stop by my place for a nightcap?"

I blinked. He certainly didn't need one and damned if I was about to share one with him.

He swung the black beast into a driveway beside a cowshed and revved the engine as he pulled up before a darkened worker's house.

"Home Sweet Home." He smiled at me and reached a hand across the car toward me. I shrank away, one hand tight on the door handle.

"No, thanks. Can you please take me home now?"

The space between his brows narrowed. "You can at least come in for a drink."

"No, thank you. I don't want one."

"Well, then, just come in and let me get a warmer jacket."

I frowned at him, then bit my lip as my heart raced. "I'll wait in the car."

"Come on, I won't hurt you. You're being silly."

Somehow, call me thick, he persuaded me to get out of the car and climb the three concrete steps to his porch. I'd barely stepped over the threshold when he wrapped his arms around me and started nuzzling my neck.

"Back off," I growled. He didn't listen, so I drove my heel into his instep and spun out of his grasp before he could respond, then reached for a handy fireplace poker.

Marcus froze and stared at my, or rather his, weapon. He suddenly seemed acutely sober. Only his Adams apple moved as he swallowed hard. Seems he wasn't game to try again and he took a deep breath.

"I'll give you a ride home," he said, his words barely audible and his eyes not quite meeting mine.

"I'd rather walk," I said, and stepped unchallenged past him and out the door. I held onto the poker until I was well out of his driveway, then threw it back toward his mailbox.

Wondering why I'd been stupid enough to wear heels, I kicked them off and started walking north. It should only be about three kilometers to home—nearly long enough to cool off. For now, I let the expletives fly at full noise. There was no one out here but the roadside cows. They didn't seem bothered—in fact, they came to the fence to stare.

Few people driving along the road could be worse than the idiot I'd just left, so I walked on, stomping my bare feet as much as the tar-sealed road would allow.

Unfortunately for Moira, my mood hadn't improved by the time I reached her on the phone early the next morning. I suspect she won't try to set me up again.

By Monday morning, my attitude had improved, thanks to Sunday's half-tub of Tip Top chocolate ice cream (even that cowshed didn't rate next to Marcus, it seemed) and I showed up at the clinic bright and early.

Karen lifted a hand to me and returned to her telephone call. No one else was in yet, so I picked up my call list for the day. No farm visits until ten.

Good.

The pile of incomplete farm call sheets and patient records on my desk took up an ominous amount of space. Almost as much space as my dead monitor—the one I brought with me from the States. Its 110-240 volt switch on the back worked, but it seems the input still had to be only 110 volts, not 230. One glorious burst of brilliant illumination, then the screen squealed to its black death, never to light up again. I really did need to get rid of it.

Line Two rang and a glance over to Karen's desk showed she was still on another call.

I bit my lip for a moment, then decided I had to answer it.

"Hello, Te Awamutu Animal Medical Center," I said, as cheerily as possible, given my terror of what I guessed was to come.

"Hi, this is *mumble, mumble, mumble* from out *mumble mumble*. I have three cows with *mumble mumble*."

I took a deep breath. I hadn't been in New Zealand very long and some of the local farmers spoke a strain of Kiwi that passed for English, but completely eluded me over the telephone. I could decipher some of these men's meaning by watching their mouths and hands in person, but on the phone, all bets were off.

"Hello, have I lost you?" came the voice on the other end.

"Ahh… no, sorry, I'm here. Must be a bad line. Could you please repeat that? I didn't get it all." Or any of it, actually, but he didn't need to know that.

Same answer. Couldn't even get the name after I asked him to speak more slowly. *Twice* more.

After his final attempt, I was ready to smack my forehead on the desk and he sounded more than a little annoyed.

A flood of relief washed over me as I noticed Karen hovering beside me.

"One moment please, sir," I managed with a strangled cry and thrust the phone at the ever-efficient office manager.

She smiled, but a twitch had started up at the corner of one eye as she grabbed for the phone. All professionalism, she took the call. "Hello, Karen here, may I help you?"

I took a deep breath to attempt to regain some equanimity while I listened.

"Ahh, Mr. Peabody-James, you have three cows to be cleaned? Out at your Paterangi runoff? Excellent," she muttered, scuttling sideways to the daybook she ruled with an iron fist. "And no, we won't send her. Jarrod Woodsley will be there at 10 a.m. if it suits? Wonderful. Thank you for your call." She rang off and winced. "He does speak rather fast," she said, and chuckled.

"With a mouthful of marbles, I suspect," I said beneath my breath as my face heated.

"You'll get used to it." Karen didn't sound convinced.

Wondering how long it would take, I gave thanks my horse clients spoke the good Queen's English. Luckily, I had mostly horse clients, as I was the one horse vet to the eight dairy vets in our practice. I was hard-pressed to learn about cows during my first "calving season" when I first joined the group.

Upon hiring me earlier in the year during my very first New Zealand vacation, I wondered why my new boss had told me to "go on home to California and sell up. Just make sure you're here by the first of July."

I clearly didn't understand the ramifications of that sentence.

I must have had some mental image of waltzing with smiling Jersey cows through fields of daffodils as the days gave way to balmy summer temperatures. I *knew* the seasons were reversed, but that minor detail had somehow slipped my mind.

I flew into Auckland on the first of July to torrential rain—rain that barely let up for the next three months—and a cloud cover that only lifted for a few hours each afternoon, *if* you were lucky.

Cows in the mud, anyone?

"So what would you like for Christmas?" Karen's voice brought me back to the present. She smiled as she handed me the on-call schedule for the next three months, including the Christmas holidays. "Surprise! Early bird gets the worm. You're off from Christmas to New Year's!"

"Thanks, that's a pretty nice Christmas present," I said with a smile, but I felt a little empty inside. It wasn't what I *really* wanted for the holiday, but it seemed this would have to do. With no family in New Zealand, I wasn't even sure what I was going to *do* for the holiday, but I'd find something. Having survived one Waikato winter and springtime, I'd surely earned my summertime Christmas, like the one pictured so vividly on the pages of my *New Zealand the Beautiful Cookbook*: sun-bronzed kids on the beach against a backdrop of sailboats, a glittering sea, and scarlet-flowering Pohutakawa trees, with the luscious Kiwi summertime holiday fare spread out before them.

It sounded a lot more fun than shoveling snow. And I'd done enough of that to last me a lifetime.

After a particularly hellish day one week later — defined by this horse vet as a full day of pregnancy testing cows—I'd finally gotten blessedly clean, though I'd probably be green-stained and smell like cow manure forever. Luckily, Moira wouldn't care.

Tomorrow, she and I were going out to the movies—she said she owed me, and I didn't disagree. I needed a good night out—without drunken louts.

I was snuggled warm under my goose-down duvet when the jangle of the phone in my ear jerked me from my pleasant stupor. I wasn't on call, but my body didn't know that… and the effect was the same, either way. One deep breath to still my jumping nerves as I struggled to a sitting position, then I picked up.

"Hello, Marcus Madsen here. Look, I wondered if you'd like to—umm—well, I just wanted to apologize. Sorry about last week. I don't know what came over me."

It must be getting close to date night.

"It was probably all the booze you drank." I *may* have spoken a bit tersely.

"Yes, that was it," he said, with palpable relief in his voice. "So, would you like to try again? Saturday, there's a party—"

"You're blaming your behavior on the alcohol? Now I've heard everything." I snorted, then laughed outright.

"Ahh…" Silence. "I'm not usually—"

"Look, Marcus, you may not go to church, but does the phrase 'a cold day in Hell' mean anything to you?"

"Ahh…"

"Forget it. You've melted your brains. First off, didn't your mother ever tell you not to ring people at this hour? Second, the answer is no. And it always will be. I don't do drunks. I certainly don't do drunk drivers. Good *night*," I growled, and slammed the phone down onto the receiver with relish.

Despite my late-night wind up, I was somewhere past exhaustion, so sleep pulled me under the minute I lay back down. With a smile on my face.

3

I'd injected the final cow in John Munro's cowshed when I saw an old girl standing in the paddock next to the vet race.

"What's with her, Mr. Munro?"

"She's been dragging her toes... barely moving around since she calved and she's off her tucker," he said, glancing away.

"She hasn't been eating much while I've been here," I murmured. The Jersey stood in knee-deep grass, but none of it near her appeared to have been touched.

"Nope, she hasn't really eaten in two days," he said, "and I filled that water bucket beside her last night. She hasn't had a drop."

I swallowed hard. Not a good look, but I'd seen worse.

"She's been a good 'un." He blinked a few times, then drew his sleeve across his eyes and shook his head, staring away from me out across the paddocks.

The ancient Jersey raised her head and gave him a long

look, then dropped it again to rub her muzzle on one fetlock, but still she didn't eat.

"How old is she?" The cow seemed to hold the knowledge of the world in her big, soft eyes.

"Last count, nineteen." He swallowed hard. "She's calved every year, usually a heifer."

"So why is she up here?" I said, a sick feeling growing in the pit of my stomach.

The farmer winced and glanced at the shiny black car sitting in the cowshed roundabout. "Madsen. He'll be back up here at the shed soon."

I flinched at Marcus' name. I'd parked right next to a black Holden, but in my hurry, I hadn't recognized it as his.

I frowned. "We might be able to help that cow, if you're not ready to let her go yet."

His eyes shot to my face. Hope leapt in them for a moment before the shutters slammed closed and he looked at the ground again. "Nobody's been able to fix 'em before. You just spend more money before they have to go on the truck," he muttered.

I hesitated before answering. Some of these older farmers were tough nuts to crack with unfamiliar therapies. "As long as her pelvis isn't fractured, acupuncture should help her"—I looked away myself now, from the crusty old cow cocky's glistening eyes—"and that paresis, the weakness, in her hind end should go away soon."

He jerked his eyes up from their study of his gumboots. "Really?" He straightened up and took a deep breath. "Nobody's done that before on this place."

"Most vets around here haven't had the opportunity to

learn acupuncture yet, but I have. It's the best thing for these cows."

"Hey, John!" came Madsen's voice from around the front of the shed.

"We're in here," he said, and gritted his teeth.

The agent's slicked-back hair shined around the corner and he nodded at me. "Mornin, miss, um"—his voice trailed off as he recognised me—"Doc."

I raised a brow and nodded back. "Mr. Madsen," I said through tight lips. The steely gaze I shot at him was safer than the words trying to scream their way out of my mouth.

Marcus gulped and turned back to John. "We're takin' that old screw too, right?" He waved his biro at the doe-eyed cow.

John looked at me and I shook my head, trying to keep the triumph from showing on my face.

"Nope," he said.

The stock agent's brows narrowed for a moment. "Well, I'll be off then," he said to no one in particular, and soon the glistening jet SRV raced away, enveloped in a cloud of dust. Hopefully, covered with it.

John and I turned back to the cow.

"Please, Doc, if you can do anything for her, I'd sure appreciate it," he said, his face hidden from me. He snuffled a little as I went back to the vat room to wash up and get my needles.

The lovely old Jersey stood like a rock in the middle of the paddock while I placed her acupuncture needles. The only restraint we needed was the farmer's hand scratching her ears and behind her horn nubs. She breathed softly, her eyes closed as she rubbed against John's hand until she fell asleep with the needles in her.

She roused long enough to lift her head and drink half of her bucket of water. John was nearly bouncing with delight. "It's turning her around!"

I nodded and smiled, then continued placing her needles.

"Can you keep her out of the herd?" I said when I'd finished, as I snapped my bag closed.

"She can stay in here." His reply was instantaneous. He'd clearly already decided this.

I smiled.

In the vat room, he handed me a pristine, white scrubbing brush and the near-boiling water hose to wash my boots. "You coming in? The missus has new feijoa jam and a leg of hogget for lunch."

"Don't mind if I do." I grinned up at him. "Thank you, John. I hear your wife makes the best hogget in the district."

"Who says *that*?" He peered sideways as he led the way to the house.

"My boss."

"Ah, of course… the fine Mr. Harrington. Yes, I imagine he does. Funny how his visits are always right on lunchtime." His eyes danced. "Thanks to you, we've got something to celebrate today."

I winced. "She looks better, but let's not count our chickens yet."

He motioned me to precede him up the back steps to the washroom. "Sara," he called out through the open back door as he kicked off his gumboots, "I've brought the new lady vet up for lunch."

Mrs. Munro introduced herself at the back door and welcomed me. She was a tall, buxom brunette who managed to look a lady, even in her farm attire. I followed her up the back stairs, left my boots in the washroom, and stepped into the big farmhouse kitchen.

"Mrs. Munro, thanks for having me to lunch," I said, then froze in my tracks.

A veritable feast was laid out on the massive kitchen table. The old totara table took up half of the oversized room, crowned by its enameled Aga built into the far wall. The gorgeous old stove was big enough to roast the whole leg of hogget, which took pride of place in the middle of the spread. "Ah, I don't mean to intrude if you're having a party today."

"Party? Oh no," she laughed, "this is just regular, everyday lunch. The boys get hungry. They'll be up in a few minutes. They know we have company—and they're taking their sweet time scrubbing up." She chuckled at her husband, then stifled her mirth as she turned to me. "Would you like to use my bathroom to tidy up? It's a lot cleaner. Third door on the left." She gestured down the hallway. "And please, call me Sara."

"Thank you," I said, and turned in time to see him walk in the door.

He had to be Sara's son: same eyes, hair and height. As he glanced my way, molten chocolate eyes melted into mine and I was caught. I found my mouth was open and hurriedly slapped it shut. He looked vaguely familiar, but I couldn't remember where I'd seen him before. Maybe in some dream.

As if from far away, Sara's voice came to me. "Nigel, this is Lena. She's the new vet at Harrington's practice."

"Ah, so finally we meet, officially," he murmured. "I've heard so much about you." He, at least, could speak—and smoothly at that. Nigel reached for my hand and I remembered to offer it and shake in return. "I guess this is how you greet a lady vet?" He hesitated for a moment, then continued. "You warned me against getting too close the last time." Nigel chuckled.

I must've been smiling like an idiot, my face hot, but then I remembered where I'd seen him before. The room wobbled a little and I took a deep breath to steady myself.

Oh no... it isn't possible... but yes, it is.

Somerfield's cowshed.

With the realization, I wanted to crawl into a hole, but I somehow managed to extricate my hand and drop my gaze to the floor.

"You scrub up okay," he said, his voice warm. "You'd clearly had a rough day when I met you. And you smell so much better today."

I quickly glanced up into his face again, but saw nothing but approval and kindness.

His face and muscular arms were tanned, as was the rest of him, or whatever skin showed around the edges of his tight, black wool shearing singlet and rugger shorts—plenty. I swallowed and averted my eyes before I embarrassed myself any further.

"I was just going to wash up," I murmured at my socks

and escaped down the hall. Locating the promised bathroom, I slid the bolt across and leaned back against the door, breathing more quickly than a walk down the hall should've engendered. When I finally opened my eyes, I stared straight at my flushed reflection in the mirror.

Get a grip, girl, it's just a man.

But what a man.

And he still likes you, even after your first… meeting.

I washed carefully and just as carefully schooled my thoughts on the way back to the table. I loved New Zealand. Loved everything about it. It was so different from the country where I'd grown up and learned my veterinary profession, but this was the side I'd yearned for—the real farming side. And the sight of the last farmer I'd seen didn't hurt.

Not one bit.

IN ALL, THREE "BOYS" had come in.

"Lena," Nigel nodded at the other two men, "this is my brother Jake and our worker Sam."

"Nice to meet you both," I said, my wits returned.

Sam looked at me and grinned as I slid into in the chair Sara indicated. "Always wondered what a girl cow vet looked like," he said.

"Well, actually a horse vet, but cows come with the job."

Nigel laughed. "You're the first female vet that practice's ever had." He picked up the tray of hogget from the top of the Aga and held it before me. My face heated as I gritted my teeth and forked some of the perfectly-roasted meat.

I'm twenty-eight, for goodness sake, and acting like a bloody virgin.

"Ladies can do anything now, gentlemen." Sara smiled and shook her head. "So Lena, John says you've acupunctured our Georgette."

"Georgette?" I glanced at John, who ducked his head and gulped his tea.

Nigel's mother continued in a soft voice. "She's a very special cow to us. Thank you for helping her."

An unexplained shiver ran up my spine. Something about her tone, but I could find no reason for it. "There's no evidence of a pelvic fracture," I said. "Hopefully the needles will quiet down her inflamed pelvic nerves and relieve the pain that's put her off her feed and slowed her down."

Sara looked out the window toward the cowshed yard, and a smile spread across her face. "She looks to be eating now. She hasn't really done much of that in the last few days."

"She started ripping up grass halfway through her treatment," John puffed out his chest, "and she scoffed the whole bucket of water that's been sitting there untouched for days."

Two pairs of cocoa eyes turned my way, one brimming with tears.

"She was our boy's 'calf club' calf. He loved her to bits," Sara murmured and stared at her plate.

I looked at Nigel and smiled. "Your heifer, or your brother's?" I looked from him to Jake.

Jake pressed his lips together and looked away.

"His brother's." John mumbled.

"Oh," I said, and promptly bit my lips together, as everyone silently busied themselves with lunch or their fingernails. There didn't seem to be anything else to say, but I wondered what I could've possibly said.

"Try some feijoa jam," Sara said with forced brightness. Sunlight shone through the jar's golden gem-coloured goodness as she handed it over.

Maybe I just imagined it.

The talk picked up again gradually—the incident forgotten or buried—prices at stock saleyards, girl vets, and talk of the job Nigel had recently left—managing a big station in Taumarunui.

"So my boys have both come back to run the farm and we can retire," Sara said with a sigh.

"Don't think you'll get rid of me yet, boys," John nodded in their direction and laughed.

"I'll leave that up to Mum," Nigel said, and squeezed his mother's hand on the table beside him.

They didn't seem to have even made a dent in the food by the time everyone had tucked into the not one, but two desserts—no, *puddings*, Kiwis called them—gracing the table. I wondered how Sara kept her figure. Probably by catching and cooking her own sheep for dinner and running after all these men.

I finally stood up, not sure if I'd be able to eat for the next week. "Mrs. Munro—Sara—thank you so much for having me to lunch. It was fantastic, but I need to get going to my next call. It's way out in Ngaroto."

"It's been lovely to meet you," she said, and the rest called their goodbyes as I left the room. I didn't dare meet Nigel's eyes. As I slipped into my gumboots at the bottom of the stairs and turned to wave, my hand met flesh with a resounding slap and I froze. It was Nigel's cheek. I'd caught him as he leaned forward to pull on his paddock boots.

"Oh, I'm so sorry!" I closed my eyes and straightened up, wishing the ground would just go on and swallow me. My face, hot before, positively steamed now.

His eyes danced. "Forfeit," he said, and walked away toward the cowshed and my ute.

"Forfeit?"

"Yep, forfeit. You owe me now."

I followed him, struggling to match his long stride.

"You slapped me, so I choose the forfeit," he said, with that lazy grin.

Biting my cheek, I frowned up at him. "And your choice?"

"A date, Saturday night. That is, if you're not going out with anyone." His eyes searched my face as he bit his lip, with a slight narrowing of his brows.

"Oh, no, definitely not," I said with vehemence, and glanced at his left hand.

No ring.

His sunny smile returned, but was there a shadow of something behind his eyes? I took a deep breath. Despite the attraction, I was unsure if I even *wanted* to try dating again.

Why the heck not?

"Okay," I finally said. Not all guys could be as bad as the last jerk. But then, I always said that…

As we walked on, he gazed down at me, then frowned. "You have a question."

"Two, actually. First, the easy one. Do you drink and drive?"

He looked at me in horror. "My mum would have my guts for garters, no matter my age. Absolutely not."

"Good. Thanks for that. And not so simple," I hesitated, then went on carefully, "what did I stick my foot into back there, with Georgette?"

He was silent, then he stopped and leaned against a fencepost. "My other brother…" his chest rose and fell a few times before he straightened up and looked straight at me, "was nine… when Georgette was his 'calf club' calf. He spent every waking moment with her, but when she fell into the Waikato River, over there," he pointed, "he couldn't pull her out. Determined to save her, he knotted her rope around his hand and leapt in—"

"Oh my God, Nigel," I said, as he went all blurry thorough my tears.

"The current was so strong, Dad and I couldn't get to them. Georgette eventually reached a place along the mostly-sheer riverbank where she could climb out, a kilometer or so down, but Adam had been sucked under and drowned by the time she dragged him out." He drew in a ragged breath. "But she… she brought him back to us. She's pretty special, and I thank you for giving her another chance."

He led me to my ute and opened the door, then handed

me in. I was so stunned by his revelation, I barely noticed the handkerchief he pressed into my hand.

"Until Saturday, then?" he said, his voice soft as he pulled a folded piece of paper from the pocket of his jeans. "Here's my number. Let me know where to find you."

"Yes," I said, and handed his now-damp handkerchief back to him.

"Keep it. See you soon."

I took a deep breath, squeezed the hand he offered, and drove away.

The weekend seemed a long way off—but for him, I think I could wait.

4

"How's Georgette?" I asked Nigel, as he opened the passenger door of his restored '68 SS Camaro and handed me in.

"She's looking okay," he said lightly, after he'd seated himself and the engine roared into life. He pulled away from the curb and turned the car away from town.

"I thought we were going to Hamilton," I murmured, then swallowed hard, my heart beginning to beat faster. Shadows of my last date flooded my mind as my hand squeezed tighter on the door handle.

Nigel flicked a smile at me. "We are, but I've something to show you first."

We headed south on State Highway 1 out of town and turned left at Kihikihi.

His eyes met mine as we continued on toward Arapuni, then turned right. "Don't worry, we'll be to Hamilton in time for the movies."

When he turned into his own driveway, I finally figured out what he was up to.

In the paddock beside the driveway with her head turned toward us stood Georgette, her fawn and black coat shining in the sun. We clambered out and I was so excited I started to hop over the fence, skirt or no skirt.

"Lena," Nigel called out with a shake of his head. He grinned at the opened gate beside him, then motioned me through.

Georgette's languid eyes perused us as she slowly chewed, while two calves cavorted about her in grass up to their bellies.

"Thank you," he murmured, and leaned down to kiss me. "Was that worth the drive out here?"

"Thank you for showing her to me. She looks wonderful." And she did. Georgette had gained weight and her bag swung full as she strode toward us. She nosed us both, then sidled closer so we could scratch her withers.

The rest of the evening, despite the liberal dusting of our clothes with fawn-colored Jersey hair, was pure fairytale. We drove up to Hamilton and started looking for dinner. California food snob notwithstanding, it still made me shudder to think the fourth largest city in New Zealand still sported Copp and Co. as their "finest" dining establishment. I was grateful there was a Mexican restaurant in town, no matter how anglicized its menu.

While ordering dinner, Nigel ask for a beer and I froze. He flicked a glance at me and raised a questioning brow.

I gulped, my heart pounding in my chest.

"What is it, Lena, are you okay?" He looked at me, concern in his eyes.

I took a deep breath. "I'm still a little gun-shy from my last date."

"Why, what happened?" he asked, and I told him a little about my trip to Taumarunui.

He shook his head. "You don't need to worry about that with me. I don't do things like that—any of them," he said, then leaned back in his chair and regarded me, a question in his eyes. Then he leaned toward me and reached for my hand. "I knew I'd seen you before somewhere," he said, as he nodded his head slowly.

I flicked my gaze from our linked hands up to his face. "Pardon? Where?" I closed my eyes and swallowed hard. "Other than in that disgusting cowshed."

He laughed. "Like I said before, you scrub up well. I was in that pub in Taumarunui, the one with the dinner show. Glanced through the door from the public bar into the dining room and saw the prettiest girl I'd ever seen, dressed to the nines. Sitting at a table with a loser drunk."

"You were there?" A chill began in the pit of my stomach.

"Yes. Now I wish I'd stayed a little bit longer. I wasn't keen to get in the middle of a domestic when you looked like you were handling the situation, so I didn't worry too much."

"Well, I didn't handle it very well," I growled.

"Sounds like it. So, you ended up letting him drive?"

"I couldn't get the keys off him."

Nigel shook his head. "I'd have dealt to him if I knew.

You looked to be in full control of the situation—cool and calm."

"Yeah, well, vets *have* to look like that. All the time. I should've taken the keys from him or refused to drive home with him, but shoulda, coulda, woulda. It's over now, but it hasn't endeared me to drunks. Hence my concern about a simple beer."

"Like I said," Nigel's gaze locked with mine, "it's not a problem with me. Ever. I promise you that."

CHILES RELLENOS FILLING my stomach and the sight of Nigel filling my head, we danced the night away to the live band at the RSA. We taught each other a few new moves and had a blast. Yes, he could even dance.

No better combination, bar none.

Especially after my last train wreck of a date.

Later that night, he handed me out of his car and kept hold of my hand as he led me to the door.

His lips warm against mine. Our first real kiss was all I could've asked for as we held to each other for long, warm minutes.

"Next weekend, would you like to head out to Kiritehere? I could take you out to my uncle's farm and maybe go for a swim."

"Sounds wonderful," I breathed, and took his lips again.

It'd been a long time.

"Well, good night," he said finally, drawing away with reluctance. I bit my lips together. It would be so easy to invite him… but no, not yet. Much as I'd like to, it never worked.

"Until Sunday, then," he whispered, and kissed me fleetingly once again before he turned to go.

I was still smiling as the tail lights of his Camaro flicked on, then disappeared into the night.

"HELLO, NIGEL HERE." His voice warmed me more than even my fireplace on this cold evening.

"Good to hear from you," I murmured lazily. The man sounded as keen as I felt. And it was only Wednesday.

"I said I'd see you Sunday," he said, "but I didn't want to wait that long to talk with you."

I didn't think I could get any warmer, but I was wrong.

"Nice." *Good one, Lena.* My brain clearly wasn't working, although he was twenty kilometers away. "Me, either," I managed.

"I had an actual excuse to ring, anyway. Two, actually. First, Georgette is looking well and Dad wants you to come out and treat her again. 'Just so she doesn't slip backwards,' he says."

"No problem. What else?"

"Thought if you don't mind cold water, we could go whitebaiting while we're out at the coast on Sunday."

"Ohhh, I'd love to. I've always wanted to try it, and water's no problem—I'm a fish."

He chuckled and my stomach clenched at the rumble of

his deep voice. "Sounds good. It's a date, then. Pick you up at seven a.m.? We want to make the tide."

"I'll be ready. Have a lovely week," I said wistfully.

"Ta da. See you soon," he said, and rang off.

As it turned out, Georgette *was* looking better when I visited them a few days later. Much better. Only the slightest limp remained and she continued to pick up weight. I kept catching knowing smiles between Nigel's mum and dad, but they said nothing about the blossoming relationship between their son and me.

I acupunctured Georgette again and afterward had to attend the requisite lunchtime feast. My boss was right.

Sara was amazing.

SEVEN A.M. Sunday couldn't come early enough for me. My togs and towel packed, I leapt up at the sound of his ute in the drive.

This time, kisses came first. It seemed we were on our way to starting something real.

On the long drive out to the coast, he kept taking my hand. I couldn't keep the idiot-grin from my face.

"Biscuits?" I waggled a brow at him.

"Before breakfast?" He glanced at me, brows narrowed in mock horror.

"These are healthy ones, well, maybe other than the chocolate," I said, as we exited Otorohanga, heading south.

"So, that's why you wanted some milk fresh from the vat."

"Mmmm…" I said, grinning. "Jersey milk. No better."

By the time we reached the deathtrap of a Waitomo turnoff, we'd each had several bikkies, washed down with the fresh milk.

"Though it's bad luck to eat before fishing, it's okay for whitebaiting, so I'm taking you to the hotel here for breakfast," Nigel said.

"I'll never say no to breakfast, but won't we miss the tide?"

"There is that." He looked sideways at me.

"Let's go. I've brought lunch, too."

His face glowed. "Woman after my own heart. I'd best watch out," he said, then his jaw tightened and he swallowed hard.

I looked out the windshield to see what he'd seen, but there was nothing amiss. By the time my eyes returned to his face, the shadow was gone.

Must've imagined it.

The 19th century Waitomo Caves Hotel on top of a bluff beside the road flashed past, its woodwork reminiscent of days long past.

He saw me staring up the hill. "We'll go there sometime, if you like. Nice place. Have you been to the caves?"

"I have, but only to walk through, which is pretty awe-inspiring anyway. I'd love to take one of their adventure tours with the underwater rafting, rappelling, and caving."

"Me too. We can go rappelling out in our valley." He looked away from the road briefly to give me a warm smile.

"That'd be great. I've seen people doing on those bluffs from the road."

"Yes, that's the place. Our neighbors let me use them whenever I want."

"How did I find another adventurer?" I couldn't help beaming at him.

Again. Or was it *still?*

THERAPEUTIC CHOCOLATE and Nigel's tour-guide chatter notwithstanding, by the time we'd driven the sixty-odd kilometers of roads out to the coast—roads that would make you cry if you were in a hurry and got behind one of the ever-present tourist motorhomes: tortuous, narrow, bush covered, partly tar-sealed, albeit beautiful—I was sick as a dog. I'd firmly planted my gaze on the winding goat track before us and didn't look away, but I was still ill. I'm sure it was despite, not because of, the chocolate. And I'm sticking to my story.

My stomach settled when I hit the water at Marokopa, a big, fine net in my hands. Nigel had placed me in the waist-deep tidal river beside several other whitebaiters. Their leathery, bronzed skin bespoke their enthusiasm for fishing in general and whitebaiting in particular.

"What are they, the whitebait?" I questioned Nigel. "Are they full grown?" I asked.

"They're juvenile forms of several kinds of galaxiids. We're catching them as they migrate upriver to grow. Some of them spawn up there and others come back down to estuaries to lay their eggs."

I caught one up in my hand and inspected it. "They're so tiny… doesn't seem right to eat them." Their translucent little bodies were only an inch and a half long by an eighth of an inch thick. "They wouldn't make much of a meal."

He winced. "Not individually, but cooked into an omelette—well they have to be tasted to be believed."

Poor little beggars. I'd be sure to give plenty of thanks.

"Ready to go in?" Nigel called from his position upriver after we'd been at it for three hours.

"Yes. It's wonderful being out here in the water, but I'm getting pretty stiff."

His eyes twinkled. "Most newbies don't last half as long as you did."

"So now, we make a fire and cook them?" I threw over my shoulder as I scrambled up the crumbling sandbank.

"Nothing so primitive as that." He gave me a mock frown as he took the heavy net from my stiff fingers. "We go up to my uncle's and use *his* stove. I'm sure he and old Ben will appreciate fresh fish for lunch."

"Does he know we're coming?"

"No, but we'll have hot food waiting when Don gets in for lunch," Nigel said, as he put the ice cream container, chocker with little fish, into his chilly bin.

"All prepared, aren't you?" I peered into the cooler, complete with ice, on the back of his ute.

His eyes glittered as he snapped the lid shut and took my hand. "Come here, I've missed you," he said, as he pulled me into his arms and kissed my lips.

"But we've only been a few feet apart," I protested, when we finally came up for air.

"Yeah, well, I didn't want to give those old boys out there fishing with us a heart attack."

I shook my head at him and laughed.

"Let's load these nets and get up the hill. I'm starving." He flashed me one of his molten glances. "But I want food, too," he whispered.

My knees were already melted *before* that comment. I could only take a deep breath to steady myself as I stepped back. More winding roads, straight up the hill towering high above the ocean cliffs, and we were there.

5

Kiritehere.

I suspect it was once more populated than the handful of houses there now. It was somewhere almost off the map but had the distinction of being on the sole coastal backroad from Raglan to Awakino. Two hundred kilometers of narrow, tightly-winding road. Ideal if you had several days to enjoy the gorgeous, bush-clad journey—and stomach of iron.

Before us stood a fenced yard with a small house that'd probably been there at the turn of the century. The lawn before the house was mowed, but the dwelling still looked forlorn, with only the remnants of dried-up spring bulbs lying amidst the weeds to embellish its exterior.

"My Uncle Don's place. Land of Angus cattle, Romney sheep, and steep hills." Nigel cut the engine and hopped out. Before I could untangle myself from the seatbelt, he was already there, holding the door open for me.

"I could get used to this, you'd better watch out," I said, lifting my chin for another kiss.

"That seems to be my aim." His eyes smoked. A day in cold water hadn't dampened his enthusiasm, nor mine.

I hoped I knew what I was doing, because I was falling fast.

Straightening up, I shook my head. "I can see I won't get much done around you," I said, looking past his shoulder at the sad little house. "Does your uncle live out here all alone?"

"Yes. My aunt died of cancer a few years back."

"Oh, no," I whispered.

He nodded. "She only told him about it when she was on death's door. There was nothing that could be done."

"Didn't they have any children?"

"Their two sons are long escaped to the city. This block is steep on the hills, boggy on the flats, and sandy everywhere else. It's lovely, but a hard place to survive on, much less make a living. I'm not sure what he's going to do with the place—neither of his kids wants to farm, especially not," he broke off and surveyed the precipitous, sheep-covered hill country as far as the eye could see, "way out here. It seems to be the way of it in New Zealand these days."

"So he truly *is* alone."

"Well, no." Nigel gave me the ghost of a smile. "He's got Ben."

I looked askance at him.

"Ben, his working dog. Uncle Don is my mother's eldest

brother—and he's getting on a bit. Problem is, Ben's not young, either." Nigel frowned and bit his lip, then seemed to remember I was there and squeezed my hand, tugging me toward the front door.

It opened to his touch. He stepped inside and looked around. "Uncle Don?" No one answered, so he turned and motioned me in.

"He doesn't mind us walking in like this?"

He turned to me, his brow furrowed. "He's my uncle."

"And he doesn't lock it?"

Nigel laughed and gave me a hug as he gazed down into my eyes. "There's only one road out here. We know everyone living along it and no one takes kindly to things like that. You'd be pretty stupid to steal out here." His eyes hardened. "Someone was doing the rounds during a community event when everyone was at the local hall. They later found the guy's van, full of stolen goods, but nothing else. Hasn't happened since."

I swallowed hard. It was tough to eke out a living on these hills—tough men and women. Not good people to mess with.

I gulped. "Sounds like a safe place to live, if you're not a thief."

"You'll do fine," he said, his gaze lightning. "I'll protect you."

"Who needs protecting?" said a gruff voice from the doorway, as a wet nose edged between us.

Nigel stepped back and turned to face the grizzled man at the entrance. "Uncle Don!" He went to him and threw his arms around him. "It's been a long time. I'd like you to meet Lena."

He nodded, then thrust out his hand. "Pleased to meet you," he murmured, then turned back to Nigel. "So, who needs protecting?" he repeated.

"No one, Uncle. It's all good," Nigel said, bending down to greet the even grayer black and white eye dog. "How are you goin', old man?"

Ben glanced back and forth between Nigel and Don while he submitted to Nigel's pats, then stepped lightly toward me.

"This is Lena, Ben, prettiest girl horse vet in Te Awamutu."

I quirked my lips. "I'm not sure that's much of a complement. I'm the *only* girl horse vet in Te Awamutu."

"Trust me, it'll always be a complement for you," Nigel murmured.

Ben nosed at my hand and I ducked down beside him and stroked his fine-boned face.

One last look up at his master to confirm I was okay, then Ben glued himself to my side.

"Good to see you, Nigel. It has been a while… too long. Sorry you thought you had to go so far down the line to get over—"

"It's okay, Don," Nigel cut in sharply and flicked a glance over his shoulder at me.

What was that about?

His uncle turned to me for a moment, too, then cleared his throat and continued. "Anyway, glad you're back. What brings you out here?"

"Came to see you and take Lena out for a fish."

Don's eyes lit up. "Whitebait?"

"You came home too early. We just got here. I thought it'd go easier on us if I trashed *your* kitchen making whitebait fritters instead of Mums." Nigel's glowing eyes met mine, then he headed for a cupboard and started pulling out ingredients.

Don smiled at me. "The boy knows how to make friends, eh? So you're a vet, are you? Dogs and cats?"

"Horses. The rest just go with the job."

His brows shot up. "Maybe," he looked up at me hopefully for a moment, then dropped his eyes, "but no. It's Sunday."

"Can I help you with something? I'm happy to."

"Well, it's just that…"

"What is it, Don?" Nigel frowned, peering into the fridge. "Where are the eggs?"

"Where they've always been—in the butter safe," Don said, then turned back to me. "It's the young horse. I think he's done a tendon."

"Oh, no," I said, glancing out at the steep hill farm. Not a good outlook for a horse with a bowed tendon on those steep sidelings. "Why do you think it's a tendon?"

"It's all swollen and he's nearly three-legged lame."

"When did it start?"

"He was a little off yesterday, but today he's quite bad."

"Let's look at him now. Is there time, Nigel?"

"Sure. I'll put the whitebait in the fridge."

"With my old horse full of arthritis, I need this young one for the farm."

"What about your motorbike, Uncle?"

Don snorted. "The tracks don't go everywhere on this farm. Way too steep. No wonder my sons ran for the city." He sobered, then took a deep breath. "I'm safer on a young horse than on a four-wheeler."

I shuddered. That said a lot about the farm. And this old man was out here all alone? "I thought four-wheelers were pretty stable."

Both men chuckled. "More stable than three wheelers, maybe, but all *four* wheels really do is make them roll straighter down the hills."

"Oh." I winced, as they laughed. Another glance out the open door showed me it really wasn't a laughing matter. "No wonder you'd rather ride a horse. Let's go see him."

Don led me to the barn behind his house. "Got him from over Gisborne way," he said, beaming, as he grabbed a halter and lead from a hook on the wall.

"Gisborne-bred, eh? Nice horses," I said.

And he was. The big strapping bay Clydesdale-cross stood a good sixteen and a half hands, with a chest nearly that wide. A veritable tractor. The hill-country bred stock from the Hawkes Bay region, including Gisborne, were the most surefooted and unflappable horses I'd ever met. This one was no exception.

He stood with his right front toe barely touching the ground. Don haltered the gelding and I reached out to greet him. He pricked his ears and snuffled my hand, then licked it. Satisfied, he let his ears flop again and lifted his sore hoof, then reached down to nose at it.

"You poor darlin," I murmured, as I moved to his right side and slid my hand down his leg. Sure enough, he had plenty of filling around the flexor tendons, from his suspensory ligament all the way to his hoof. He let out a big sigh when I lifted his foot, flexing the leg and holding it clear of the ground. He never moved while I palpated his tendons. None of them were painful or thickened, but the digital pulses at the back of his fetlock were pounding.

I smiled up into Don's and Nigel's worried eyes. I could do something about this, anyway.

"Don, his tendons feel fine. I think it's in his foot. Do you have a hoof knife?"

He nodded. "Do you want an apron, too?"

"Yes, please." Thank God for that—the insides of my knees had enough bruises, without adding more.

I buckled on the thick old leather apron and lifted the hoof again. A light pare over the surface of the sole and sulci revealed a black crack near his inside heel. I followed it with my knife until with one final flick of its sharp tip, the horse jerked as a stream of thick, dark gray, stinky material oozed from the small hole.

"Ah, there it is," Don said, with a satisfied grin. "Better than a tendon."

"Infinitely so," I agreed. "Have you any povidone-iodine?"

He nodded. "I set the Zip to boil when I went for the knife. I can hot-soak it while you two play in the kitchen."

"You took the words out of my mouth, Don. Do you have a boot?"

"Sure do. I'll save some clean soaking liquid for it."

"Excellent. Is he current on his tetanus?" I asked.

"Yes, luckily he was done thee months ago."

"Perfect." As the pus drained out onto the concrete floor of the shed, the horse lowered his head again and closed his eyes, then stood his whole weight on the bad hoof.

"If you can soak it twice a day for twenty minutes in the hottest iodine-water you can get your hand into and keep it covered by a boot in between, that should be all he needs," I said. I removed the apron and rolled it up, then wiped the worst of the gunk off the knife with some straw.

"Sure can. I'll put a shoe and a pad on it after it's healed up, and pop a shoe on his other front," Don said.

"Looks like he'll be a new horse soon." Nigel smiled as he reached out to take the shoeing gear.

"Thanks again," Don said. He swiped at his eyes with his sleeve, then turned back to his horse. "Thank you, Lena," he said with feeling, then turned back to the great horse. "You don't know how much this means to me," he mumbled into his mane. "I'll see you both up at the house."

I patted his shoulder and turned to go.

Outside the barn, Nigel smiled down at me and wrapped an arm around my shoulders as we walked back to the house. "You didn't need to do that, you know."

"I didn't do much."

"Tell that to the horse, or Don. You should send him an invoice, anyway."

"Can't," I said lightly. "Not meant to be working outside the practice."

He shook his head with a bemused smile and pulled me hard against his side. "You're a tough nut, you know?"

"I've heard it said. So, tell me about whitebait fritters…" I said, and his attention turned.

6

The fritters were a success. Eggy batter, with edges fried crispy brown in butter, enveloped the tiny fish. The hundred or so tiny eyes were a bit disconcerting, but their crunchy, salty taste was exquisite.

Don couldn't be happier. His precious horse was on the mend and he loved whitebait fritters. Ben, however, was in ecstasy with a new friend to latch on to on top of the fish. Once I sat down, his grizzled chin never lifted from my thigh until Nigel mentioned the word "bike".

His head shot up, floppy-tipped ears pointed at Nigel. He stared at him with an expectancy only a heading dog could hope to match—every muscle tensed, ready for action.

"Okay," Nigel said quickly and Ben was out the door, gone in a flash of black, white, and grey.

"He's gettin' pretty stiff, but he can still move." Don's mouth worked and he looked away for a moment. When he turned back to us, his eyes were watering. "He's coming home so sore lately, I'm tempted to leave him home, but he hates bein' left behind. Howls the place down the whole time. I haven't the heart to do it to him again."

"The old boy's onto a pretty good thing here—getting to stay in at night," Nigel said, as he got to his feet. "We'd best get out there or he might move all the sheep by himself."

"Let you in on a secret, you two," Don said with a twist of his lips, "as long as you don't tell anyone. I'm already the laughing stock of the district, lettin' that dog stay in the house." Don's eyes were merry. "He even sleeps on my bed. He's partial to your Auntie's pillow, not that she'd have shared," he winced, "but I'm sure she'd be pleased we both have the comfort of another soul at night."

"I didn't know your wife, Don, but I'm sure she'd be glad of it. And that's probably why Ben can still get around like he does at his age."

"Let's go for a ride," Nigel said, taking my hand. "You can ride 'Big Red', the Honda. Have you ever ridden a bike?"

"I rode a dirt bike in my teens and loved it."

"It shouldn't take you long to figure this one out, then. Similar gears, only easier."

Big Red was a bit of a monster, and it'd been years since I had a motorbike between my knees. I was slightly terrified, but it was still fun. "I like two wheeled motorcycles better—much easier to turn," I shouted to Don. He stood beside Nigel, who was mounted on a Yamaha in the center of the small, flat paddock behind Don's house.

Nigel was laughing as I hauled on the handlebars to get it around the last corner and rode back to them. "It'll turn just fine when you're going fast."

I smiled, then sobered. I couldn't get up much speed in this paddock—and this was the only level ground in sight. I shivered as my stomach got that funny feeling. He couldn't possibly think I'd be riding it on the steep tracks leading down into the valley below?

"Ready to go?" Nigel said, as Don started walking back to the house.

"Go?"

"Down the back of the farm. Don has to wait for a truck, but we can take the bikes."

I blinked. "Ahh"— I took in the sheer cliffs making up most of the farm. "Is-is there a track?" I swallowed hard.

"Of sorts." His eyes sparkled at me. "You'll do fine. Let's go."

My mouth dried at the sight of Nigel's "track". A narrow strip of steepness, akin to a goat track, had been cut away from the side of a steep sideling—with what, I have no idea—leaving a sheer bank to the left and… a nearly vertical drop to the rocky stream bed at the bottom of the hill. I finally found my voice. "Nigel, I can't… I've never…"

"You'll be fine," he said, the corners of his mouth lifting as he reached out a hand to squeeze mine on the handlebar. "Just follow. Toot the horn if you need me to stop."

Any other objections I may've had were drowned by the sound of his Yamaha revving off and down the path before me.

Certainly I can do this.

I turned the engine on again and flicked the brake off. With a deep breath, I hit the throttle and buzzed off with my heart somewhere near my tonsils.

Couldn't I just shut my eyes?

Nigel was already far ahead as I snail-crawled down the sorry excuse for a track. Sure it was plenty wide—for sheep, maybe two abreast and crowding each other toward the bank. At a stretch, a horse. A steady, well behaved one.

I swallowed hard.

As I began to take control of the four or five horses bouncing down the trail between my knees, I started noticing the mountains in the distance and the sheep scuttling off said trail. The ewes bleated at their lambs, who ignored them and scattered, bucking around on the nearly vertical face before me. I daren't turn to look at the view behind me.

The bike soon began to listen to my slightest whim and I began to smile.

"It really wasn't as narrow as I thought." I said, quirking my lips, when Nigel stopped to wait for me at a wide spot on an open ridge. "It just looks like such a long drop on the downhill side."

"It does, doesn't it?" He chuckled. "You've done just fine. The sea air suits you." He leaned across and kissed me. "We'll have to borrow some horses next time. You'd like that better, eh?"

"I don't mind the bike now. This bike and I—we have an understanding," I said as I tore my eyes from his and surveyed the farm spread out before us. To my right, a wooden bar topped the fence wires between two fenceposts and the top two high-tensile wires were tacked down level with the third one from the top. "Is that a spar? For hunting?"

"Sure is, the Kingson Hunt rides up here from time to time."

"On this steep land?"

"Yep." He caught my eye and held it. "Where do you think our Olympians come from? This is the sort of place they begin."

"What a way to start!" One couldn't help but be impressed.

"I love it out here." Nigel's voice was husky as he stared off into the distance across the valleys below. "My mother was born on this farm."

"But you've got your home farm in Te Awamutu?"

"Yes, but this place seems to call to me."

I nodded. "Its immensity and wildness"—I slowly filled my lungs—"it gets me, too." Our gazes locked for a long moment, then I followed as he led off again.

We detoured from the main track to check troughs on our way across the farm, but Nigel finally stopped his bike and cut the engine. I rode up beside him.

"Care for some afternoon tea, milady?" He half-bowed and gestured toward a narrow gully ahead.

"Afternoon tea? Here?"

He laughed and tugged a wicker basket from its bungees on the front rack of his bike.

"I never even saw that." I chuckled.

"You were too busy gulping air to see much. What'd I tell you? You needn't have worried about the bike, you did fine. Uphill's easier, but forget about that now. Come on."

"Where now, Casanova?" I asked, as I slid from the saddle of my bike.

"You'll see," he said, mystery in his voice. A soft roaring sound in the distance became louder as we walked beside the tinkling stream running through the little valley .

"Wait here," he said, seating me on a moss-covered log, "and close your eyes.

I played along and sat, my heart beating faster as I waited. The roaring sound seemed louder now and the tiny cheep-cheeps of native Fantails, *piwakawaka*, sounded all around me. I sucked in air between my pursed lips in a fair imitation of their peeps and they flew so close I felt the breeze of their passing. I always swore they wanted to play with me, though most Kiwis told me the birds just wanted to eat the insects I scared up for them.

Senses heightened with my closed eyes, my skin tingled at the soft crunching sound of the trail beneath Nigel's boots as he returned. He didn't say a word, but soon his lips were soft on the back of my neck, then on my own lips.

"You can open your eyes now."

His glowed into mine as he took my hand and led me around the next bend.

And froze at the sight.

The ocean spread out before me, its surface a sea of glittering diamonds—a beautiful backdrop for the veritable feast spread out on a tartan picnic blanket.

It must run in the family.

I shook my head and turned to Nigel. "You did… all this?"

He smiled and led me to my place. Crystal glasses, sparkling cider, and the inevitable thermos of tea.

"Biscuits?" He opened a tin to show the ANZAC biscuits inside.

"You *made* these?"

"Well, no." He had the grace to look sheepish. "Mum's contribution, though I did the mutton."

"Good job, Nigel." I gazed over the spread again and stood on tiptoe to kiss him. "Thank you. After my near-death experience up there, it's a wonderful reward."

He stared and his hand stopped stock-still on its way to the buttered rolls. "Were you genuinely scared?"

"Actually, scared stiff, until I got my hand in, but then it was fun."

"Oh, good," he said, and resumed his creation of a filled roll. "Roll?"

"Yes, please. It smells heavenly. I didn't think I could possibly eat after our huge lunch. Must be the sea air."

He grinned and started on his own sandwich.

We ate until we could eat no more, then I lay down on the blanket beside him.

"You know," Nigel's fingers entwined with mine, "I could get used to this," he murmured.

"Me too. I haven't felt so sated—"

As I spoke, Nigel shot up to a sitting position facing away from me, every muscle taut, poised to bolt. I climbed up to my knees, eyeing our surroundings for any sign of danger, but other than a few Fantails, nothing moved.

"What's the matter?"

"Nothing," he said, as he stared off into the distance.

I watched him for a few moments, then turned away and made myself as comfortable as I could with the alarm bells going off in my head.

Another commit-o-phobe, eh? I'd had enough of those to last me a lifetime. *Please, not again.*

When I glanced back at him, he looked up and smiled.

"Ready to go?" he asked, his voice overly bright.

I glanced at him from the corners of my eyes, but he wasn't looking my way. We packed it all up, loaded the basket, and set off—without one touch.

Disappointing, at best.

I wouldn't think about the term *devastation*. I'd leave it for now. Surely he'd show his cards sometime soon.

Then I'd know what was really up.

7

"Enjoy that?" Don roared over the bikes when we arrived back at his yard.

"Sure did," I said, after I stopped my engine.

"You should've seen her—like she'd ridden a bike every day of her life," Nigel said, and pecked me on the cheek.

I slapped my mouth shut from where it was hanging while I stared after him.

The man was a yo-yo.

Maybe I was reading too much into it. Probably. I'd been known to do it before. Too many times.

"Oh, Lena," Don piped up, "Ngaire stopped by. She's with the Kingson Hunt and they're having a hunt out on their farm next weekend. They have extra horses fitted up and she wondered if you two would like to ride with them?"

Sounds like a bit of me.

"I've heard of them," I said. "I hear they're pretty wild and ride any country under any conditions—at speed."

Nigel's eyes lit up and he grinned. "Yep."

"I'll check my on-call schedule and let you guys know," I said, my heart beating faster. "I haven't had the chance to ride since I left the States and I sure miss it."

"We'll ride before then, if you'd like," Nigel said. "I'm sure Mum won't mind if we take a few of ours out around the farm. They're not very fit, but at least you can get on a horse before you go out hunting."

Then I remembered. I'd only been thinking of the galloping. "Hunting over wire?" I winced.

"Yes, 'full-wire', but there are always gates if you don't want to jump, and some fences are sparred, as you saw up the top."

I shuddered. "All the fences we hunted over on the East Coast of the U.S. were either wooden or sparred." It made my heart stop to even think of jumping wire fences.

"Our horses are used to it."

"As a vet, it still terrifies me."

Nigel's eyes sparkled. "You'll be amazed at our mounts, then."

"I'm sure I will. For a country the size of New Zealand, our Olympic equestrian teams certainly exceed expectation."

Don grinned at Nigel. "George has offered Lena their stallion to ride."

"A stallion, on the hunt field?" My jaw dropped.

"He's the coolest cucumber of the lot. Full Clyde, but the New Zealand type. Much lighter than the beer-dray draft horses you're used to from the States."

I laughed. "The Clydesdales I'm used to could *step* over the fences."

"Well, this one jumps like a stag."

This I couldn't *wait* to see.

Ben nosed his way under my hand, looking for a pat. I sat on a handy anvil mounted on a stump and ensconced his grizzled muzzle between my fingers. He gazed up with adoration, his slim body swaying with the slowly waving tail. Every few moments he peered at Don. Checking up.

I was glad the old man had someone looking after him, even if the dog was as aged as he was.

Don stood up and with a quick slip of Ben's tongue on my hand, he bolted to his master's side, ready for anything.

Nigel stood, too. "We'd best be going, Don, but it's been wonderful to see you. Thank you.

"Any time, you two. See you next weekend?"

THE WEEK FLEW BY. I'd made a few acquaintances who hunted and asked them about New Zealand hunting etiquette. Thankfully, I found it differed little from the hunts with which I'd ridden in the States.

Wednesday turned out to be a lovely day and Nigel and I met at the farm after work for a ride. Mounted on Sara's sensible Welsh Cob with Nigel beside me on his big East Coast horse, we rode over the hundreds of rolling acres filled with sheep, Angus, and their small Jersey herd. On the way home, we popped over a few fences. To my relief, my six-month hiatus from riding was as if it'd never been.

"Do you need any clothes for the hunt?" Nigel asked.

"I brought my riding clothes from the states, so I'm good, thanks, other than being totally unfit for riding."

He laughed. "I am, too. You'll be fine on Saturday, by the way. I wouldn't put you up on Jake if he wasn't completely trustworthy."

"Jake?"

"George's stallion."

"Oh." I frowned. "The weather's looking bad for the rest of the week." I gazed up at the darkening skies.

"Should stop by Saturday."

"Won't it be slippery?" I said, my voice sounding small to my own ears. Hunting anywhere, under any conditions, sounded great last weekend—but the reality was beginning to hit me.

He sighed. "It'll be fine. My advice? If things get scary, shut your eyes, give him his head, and stay balanced. Let Jake manage it. He's grown up on these hills and the horses do pretty well out there, despite our interference."

Somehow that wasn't a huge comfort.

Thankfully, back in the home paddock, Georgette waited. And she *was* a comfort. The cow looked wonderful and her two calves cavorted about her while she placidly gazed at me over the sea of grass in her private palace paddock.

"She fell on her feet, didn't she?" Nigel caught my eye.

I nodded as he nudged his horse closer, closing the distance between us, then took my hand and didn't let go until it was time to dismount.

Later, he opened my ute door and handed me in, then

kissed me before closing me in. "I'll pick you up at six on Saturday morning, then?"

"I'll be ready." I'm sure I was glowing.

The man was definitely confusing, but he seemed to be over whatever it was. It seemed we were back *on*...

Whatever that meant.

"Sorry, couldn't wait 'till the weekend to see you again." Nigel's voice flowed smooth as silk across the phone line just after I arrived home from work on Thursday.

"Six a.m. Saturday not soon enough, eh?"

"Nope."

"I'd have to agree with you." I chuckled. "What are we to do about it, then?"

"They do a nice flame-grilled steak over at Lake Karapiro."

"Karapiro?" I snorted. "There's nothing out there but farms."

"Oh ye of little faith. Pick you up in an hour?"

"Want me to bring anything?"

"Nope, just yourself."

I shook my head as I hung up the phone.

By the time he arrived, I still had no idea how we were to get steak in the middle of nowhere. And he wouldn't tell me on the half-hour to Karapiro.

"There are faster ways, but I like this one," he said, as he took my hand. His eyes sparkled at me briefly, then returned to the road. We crossed over the old one-way bridge over the hydro dam, then took the main road south. After another two kilometers, we turned off toward the lake.

"Where the heck are we going?" I couldn't help asking. We were getting further and further from civilization.

He drove off the narrow road into a wide turnout on the edge of the lake and cut the engine.

I shook my head and smiled as he hopped out, slammed his door and scooted around to open mine.

"Your dinner awaits, madame."

I looked all around me before placing my hand in his and climbing out into the balmy evening.

Nigel opened the tailgate. He flicked off the bungees holding the tarp down over the back of his ute, revealing a big red esky.

"Here, you take a handle?" he said, sliding the cooler off the truck bed.

I finally got it.

"Cool, a picnic! Perfect." I beamed at him.

"I figured we might as well take advantage of the good weather."

We carried the ice chest around the edge of the lake to a secluded area under a shady tree.

"What can I do?" I asked, as he pumped up a little folding backpacking stove.

"There's a picnic blanket in there." He grinned. "You could set up our fine dining establishment, if you would, please."

I shook out the blanket and laid the tableware he'd expertly packed while he chopped garlic and crushed peppercorns. The incredible scents wafting from his spices made me realize how hungry I was.

The man could cook.

In no time at all, he'd flash-steamed some veggies and handed me the pot. Only minutes later, when I'd just finished plating up the greens, our garlicky pepper steak hissed into the pan.

"Madame?" He cocked a brow at me.

I couldn't help shaking my head. "Medium rare, please. Charred."

"Excellent. Just the way I like it. Leaves some respect for the meat. Never could stand killing meat twice."

And excellent, it was.

"That was exquisite, Nigel," I said as he moved toward me and took my lips with his.

"You like that?" He waved around our impromptu campsite.

"Absolutely. What a perfect night."

"Mmm… I'm glad." His eyes glowed as he leaned over me again in the deepening twilight and bent his head to kiss me again.

"Wherever did you learn to cook like that?"

He stiffened and sat up, not looking at me. "It doesn't matter," he said gruffly.

"No, it doesn't," I whispered, and he turned back to face me with the ghost of a smile, then took me in his arms and kissed me until I forgot my question—and his lack of an answer.

As darkness fell, so did the temperature. Soon even our ardent kisses weren't enough to keep us warm.

"Shall we go?" Nigel sounded disappointed.

"Since there's only one blanket and I suspect you start work even earlier than I do, it's probably a good idea." I kissed him once more for good measure and sat up.

It was warm in his ute—my legs from the incredible heater in his diesel wagon, and my heart from his kisses and his warm grip on my hand.

FRIDAY'S RAINSTORMS boded no good for the Saturday hunt, but when I queried Nigel on the phone on Friday night, he only laughed.

"They'll hunt in a downpour. On vertical sidelings."

I gulped. *On a horse I'd never seen before.* A stallion, for Pete's sake.

"You'll be fine. Just remember what I told you. Shut your eyes, give the beast his head, and stay balanced."

8

I tried to remember Nigel's words of wisdom as the massive bay Clydesdale half-slid, half-bounded down the steep face of a hill just behind the master, who rode just behind the pack of hounds and the whip.

The fact this horse was often ridden by the whip didn't help much. He was used to being in front of the master and I had all I could do to keep him behind the red coat before me.

As the hounds ran baying at full cry, Jake got away from me, his reins slipping through my slithering gloves. I cursed myself for wearing leather—not string—gloves. String gloves wouldn't have slipped. With 17 hands of bolting light draught horse beneath me, I was trying to climb up my reins, eyes tearing from the strands of mane blowing back in my face, when I saw the fence. We were ten strides out, then five, then three.

I gave up trying to rate him and just balanced myself.

Thankfully, because two full strides out, he left the

ground. As we flew from a good twenty feet back, the slow motion effect let me take in the stunned, frozen faces of the riders around us as they pulled up their mounts to watch the carnage about to unfold before them. Sure I was about to die when we hit the full-wire fence, I held my breath and kept my eyes up between his perky little—much too little for a Clydesdale, I remember thinking, ridiculously—ears.

Somehow, against all odds, we cleared it, but—not surprisingly—I was unbalanced when his platter feet hit the ground again and I landed on the pommel of the saddle. Painful, but worlds better than what could have happened—or if I'd been male.

Jake threw in a few bucks, just because he could, and slowed in response to my tugging on one rein.

"You bloody beast," I murmured into his mane, as I hugged his neck, when we'd finally stopped, "you great wonderful beast, but what a bloody big jump you've got."

He snorted and dropped his head to graze and I nearly fell off over his neck.

"Oh God, Lena, I thought you were dead," Nigel said, as he slid from his Thoroughbred's saddle and ran to my side.

Jake eyed him but never lifted his head from the grass.

"What a jump," I said, my voice—and the rest of me—quivering as I looked up to see Nigel's face, blanched white beneath his tan.

"Let's not see it again, okay?" Nigel reached one hand to take mine after he took Jake's reins in the other.

"What a good idea." I took a deep breath and held it as we moved aside so the field could pass.

"I'll ride him if you want," Nigel said.

"No, it'll be fine. He's had his blat and I'll hold on better next time."

"Sure footed or no," Nigel growled, "that's the last time I put you on the whip's horse. I didn't know George was a whip now."

"Amen to that," I said, shaking my head.

JAKE WAS a perfect gentleman the rest of the day.

"Guess he needed to let me know what he could do," I said to a contrite George.

"I'm so sorry," he said, for the hundredth time. "He never does that with me."

I laughed outright and laid my arm along his on the table of the wee Te Anga Pub. "George, see any difference?" I fluttered my lashes at him.

"Ah, a bit more muscle, aye?" He laughed as he picked up his beer and stood up to leave. "I'll see you two soon, eh?"

"Yes, thanks again for the loan of the horses," Nigel said, and I echoed him, watching as he moved away to speak with someone else.

"I'm just glad you're okay," Nigel gripped my hand tighter under the table. "Plus, my mum would kill me if I'd gotten you hurt. She rather likes the new girl vet."

We'd already taken George's horses home and set them up for the night, but the horses of the non-local hunt members still stood in their massive horse trucks outside the tavern, a long line of them stretching down the road.

"They're all going home tonight?" I murmured to my partner.

He nodded and followed my eyes to a particularly loud and noisy man getting seriously drunk.

"He's driving his truck full of horses? Like *that*?"

Nigel winced. "He does it all the time."

"Over sixty kilometers of winding, almost one-way road, with a twenty tonne truck and four horses' lives at stake?" My mouth dropped open. "Surely he has a sober driver."

Nigel shook his head.

Then I took a better look around the room. He wasn't the only one. And many had already started drinking from their silver hip flasks when they were still out on the hunting field.

Suddenly it wasn't so much fun anymore.

"Can we go, please? I don't think I can watch this."

He squeezed my fingers and stood, then led me to the door. A wave to the chattering crowd and we were on our way. I shuddered for the horses in the trucks, standing and getting stiffer by the hour until it was time for their owners to finish getting drunk, then wobbling home. If they were lucky.

"I enjoyed the hunting," I answered Nigel, as he opened the ute door, "but next time, let's skip the pub?"

"You got it. Excellent idea," he said, and kissed me again.

"Dinner?" Nigel queried, as he pulled up before my flat.

"I'd love it," I said without hesitation. I'd been thinking of my empty fridge. I glanced down my filthy hunt coat and rat catcher, then shifted my gaze to the smear of dried mud coating one side of Nigel's cheek and the tiny spatters all over his neck "But we'll both need a shower first. If you have clean clothes, you could shower here"—I grinned —"but nothing of mine would fit you."

His slow smile at that idea warmed me to the tips of my toes and made my insides quiver. It must have done the same for him, by the blush suffusing his grubby face and neck.

"I-I have a change of clothes with me," he said, recovering his—shaky—aplomb.

I'm not quite sure how it happened, but we ended up in the shower—together.

Let's just say we both got squeaky clean by the time the water started going cold—and he leapt out to give me room to wash my hair in the tiny cubicle.

A kiss against the glass and his towel-dried, tanned body exited the steaming bathroom. The ring of the telephone sounded over the noise of the water.

"Want me to get that?" Nigel called.

"Please," I said. I finished rinsing my hair and opened the door a crack to grab my towel. Nigel's voice, raised, came from the other room.

Who could that be?

I hurried to dry myself and wrap a towel around me. I

entered the kitchen at a trot to see a red-faced, scowling Nigel holding the phone receiver out toward me.

Whoever could it be?

"Hello?" I said, but the phone was dead. "Who was it?"

"Said he was your boyfriend." Nigel's voice was cold. "Rather nasty about it, too. Told me to piss off."

I jerked toward him. "Who? I don't have a boyfriend—other than you, maybe. I'm certainly not going out with anyone else." My face steamed in the cool evening air coming through the open window.

"Madsen?"

"Oh," I barely stopped before I growled. "*Him.* I only went out with him once—what a mistake *that* was, but I've already told you about that."

Nigel eyed me sideways then took a deep breath and let it out slowly. He hesitated, then accepted the hand I offered.

"Now, about that dinner," he said lightly, "why don't you get dressed before I get other ideas?" He wrapped his arms around my towel-clad body for a moment, but his embrace felt… hesitant? Wooden, even?

Maybe I was just imagining it.

I sure hoped so.

"Mum and Dad invited you to come out to our bach at Kiritehere for Christmas." Nigel's deep voice warmed even my frozen hands on the phone receiver as I stood on the linoleum of my bathroom floor, water still dripping from the ends of my hair after my last vet call in the pouring rain.

"Yes, please," I managed. A flood of nostalgia engulfed me and my heart gave a jerk. "I'd love that." I missed my family and I hadn't been invited anywhere by the family of a boyfriend… well, probably since high school.

I couldn't ask for more. My Christmas wish… if I didn't mess it up somehow… might just come true.

And I couldn't wipe the idiot smile from my face.

"Can you get any time off?" Nigel asked

"I've actually been given Christmas off, right through New Year's Day. Not sure how I got so lucky, but it's rostered."

"That's fine," he murmured. "And it's not long away."

"What do I need?"

"Just your togs and clothes, really. Everything else is there."

I'd ring Sara to find out what I could contribute.

Nigel's voice dragged my wandering thoughts back. "I wondered if you'd like to meet me at the saleyard tomorrow if you're free. In your lunchtime, maybe?"

"If I can get a lunch break, I'll be there."

"Good. I'll arrive for noon. We can get some tucker."

"I'll do my level best." My grin probably went all the way through the wires.

" 'Till tomorrow, then. I'm looking forward to spending Christmas with you. Kisses," he murmured, and rang off.

I stripped off and stood under the hot shower, as warm inside from our conversation as I soon became on the outside. The glow stayed with me until I closed my eyes and knew no more.

JERSEY COWS HAVE ALWAYS BEEN my favorites, with their doe eyes and tiny cloven hooves. It always got me in trouble though, because I'd let my guard down… and the little beggars were the only cows who tended to damage me. Those wee hooves were like knives—at ninja-speed. Their bigger, slower Friesian cousins had nothin' on them.

And so I stood, leaning on the saleyard fence, wishing I had a farm so I could buy the sad-looking, thin, little calves in the pen below me and take them home. Maybe someday… maybe even soon. My heart skipped a beat, thinking of Nigel, and I checked my watch.

He should be here any minute.

Somehow, I'd managed to take a lunchtime, rather than wolfing down my food in the ute on the way to my next call.

I shivered at a sudden chill on my back and turned to see Marcus Madsen, nearly close enough to touch me. Behind him, Nigel was turning away, his dark brows almost touching. His face a storm ready to break.

Marcus reached an arm around me. Not his wisest move, but then he hadn't shown himself to be terribly bright. I twisted around and broke his hold, then slammed my elbow toward his face. I caught him in the nose, with a sickening crunch, and raced after the retreating Nigel.

"Nigel, wait!" I called, but he never turned. Plenty of

other farmers did, though, their brows lifted as they watched me run toward the parking lot. I finally caught him, just as he reached his ute.

"Nigel, what's the matter?"

The look on his face froze me to the core.

"Leaving you to your boyfriend," he snarled.

"He's *not* my boyfriend. I told you before."

"Sure looked like it, with his hand on your arse."

"He never touched my arse, though I probably just broke his nose when I saw what he was up to."

"I'm meant to believe that?" he growled low, then added, "I won't be responsible for—" He froze, then spun away, jumped into his ute and peeled out of the parking lot with a spray of metal and a cloud of dust.

The few farmers still watching the show turned away. I gazed back toward the sound of the auctioneer starting up his chant, then got into my practice ute and headed back to work.

Lunch no longer appealed.

I don't think I could eat a bite.

9

It was a long night, followed by an even longer workday. The rain never let up and I had three farms for herd pregnancy tests on my list. I tried to keep my mind on the job, but it kept wandering. By the end of the day, I was seriously wondering about my choice of careers.

No matter how many scenarios I dreamed up, I couldn't imagine how merely standing beside Madsen could have caused such a disaster. I wanted to ring Nigel and talk, but whether it was cowardice or a desire to give him time to think, I'll never know. So, I left it… and cried myself to sleep.

It'd felt so right—but now?

My blood chilled at the message on my answering machine when I returned home from work. It was Sara.

"Could you please ring me?" she said, "Nigel hasn't been home since yesterday morning and I wondered if you'd seen him?"

I flicked the machine off and rang her straight back.

"I haven't seen him today, but—" I began, then broke down in tears and told her about our meeting at the saleyard. "I have no idea why he was so upset," I finished on a whisper.

Sara gave a heavy sigh. "Would you please come out for supper?" she asked. "Maybe I can help explain."

The scenery, usually slipping by with such grandeur—the rolling Te Awamutu farmland with its hedges, the raw gray buttes of Wharepapa South—went unnoticed as I drove like an automaton toward the lovely old homestead.

"I'm glad you could join me tonight," Sara murmured.

I turned my face up to hers, my eyes spilling over once again… or was it *still*?

She took me in her arms and held me, rocking me as she must've once rocked Nigel. "The men are off at a meeting."

"Nigel?" I jerked my eyes up to meet hers.

She shook her head, her own eyes filled with tears. "I fear he's left again."

"But… why?" I couldn't keep the plea from escaping my lips.

"Come and sit down. Let's eat and then we can talk."

She pulled me to her big table, set for two. I didn't think I'd be able to eat, but it seemed to help. Afterwards, we moved to soft seats in her gracious living room before a flickering fire.

"I don't know what to do about him, myself," Sara whispered to the hands folded in her lap, then gazed up at me. "He was married to a very pretty young thing, Jamie. She was a bit flighty, but seemed to love him. Nigel was different from the man he's become—less thoughtful, more of your 'good old Kiwi rugby boy'. They were sharemilking, but he liked to go drinking with the guys and—I suspect—left her alone on the farm too often and too long."

I swallowed hard. This couldn't end well.

"One night, he came home earlier than usual and found her just coming home—in a g-string and little else. They got to fighting and he accused her of messing around on him. She left in a huff… and never came back." Sara choked on her words and sat for a moment to regain enough composure to continue. "He found her wrecked car upside down in a water-filled ditch on a straight piece of road—both her and my unborn grandchild, dead."

My world spun as I gripped Sara's hand. We cried together for their loss. I cried for their loss… and my own. This was more than I could've foreseen, or even imagined.

"Nigel left that day," Sara continued, "and we didn't hear from him for six months. Then he left a phone message to say he was alive and 'well', though he sounded far from it. We were just thankful he was alive. He said he was staying away from women and sporting clubs, but he only came home a short time before we met you over Georgette. Quite changed, he was… or so we thought… but it appears the old scars remain."

"I truly only saw that creep Madsen once—and walked two kilometers home, barefoot, to get away from him," I said in a small voice. "I adore Nigel."

Sara laughed wetly through her tears. "I know, but things are black and white for that boy. Always have been. Let's hope he sees reason. For now, I'll try to go on with my life and suggest you do the same. You're always welcome out here, remember that."

"Thank you, Sara, I appreciate you telling me all this. It makes a big difference. Please let me know if you hear anything?"

"Of course, sweetie. As soon as I hear. For now, we might not be going out to Kiritehere for the whole Christmas holidays. With Nigel back, we thought we'd be ahead on the farm jobs and could take the time, but with him gone, probably not."

"Let me know if I can help with anything."

Now she properly laughed. "You've already got a full time vet job on your hands—that's plenty."

I smiled ruefully. "True."

"We'll see how we go. If we *do* go out there, we'd love to have you. Either way, I wouldn't want you to be alone in the holidays."

I smiled a little as she hugged me and led me to the door.

It was a week until Christmas, but then suddenly it was only a few days away. I managed my grief while I was still working, but then my Christmas days off began and things, namely me, started getting a bit touchy.

I wandered the aisles of the grocery store to restock my empty cupboards, but Christmas displays bombarded me from all sides. I nearly bolted out the front door, but I truly had nothing in the house, so I buckled down and shopped. I picked out meat and veggies, plus oats, flour and sugar—I was truly out of food—and headed for the checkout.

A voice from right behind me sent shivers down my spine.

"Payback's a bitch," it whispered.

Madsen.

I didn't give him the pleasure of a response. The man was evil. The worst thing was, he probably didn't even know how *very* evil he was.

Straightening, I pushed my cart forward, willing the tears to stay back. I paid the checkout lady, then carried the bags up the block to my flat.

I had to do something. I wasn't used to being sedentary —my constitution couldn't handle it, but where could I go? I couldn't bother Sara all the time and my own family was unreachable over the holiday period.

I steadied myself and focused. Then I saw my neglected rollerblades beside the door and hugged them to my chest like an old friend.

They were a good outlet for what ailed me. For the next days, I spent most of my waking hours skating around the Te Awamutu College grounds.

The deep stillness and peace in the deserted school yards helped fill the hole in my heart. Warbling birds and the occasional sleeping neighborhood cat shared with me their pristine acres of smooth pavement and gentle ramps. The graceful curves of the netball courts let me re-perfect my figure skating. Most importantly, though, the skating let me think of something besides Nigel—even if only for an hour or two—and how I may have just wrecked his life, no matter how unintentionally.

10

Christmas Eve finally came, more slowly than it ever had before. Suffice it to say I finally made it to sleep, rubbing my sore, tear-filled eyes, wondering what I was going to do to celebrate the big day.

I didn't have long to wonder. The phone jangled me awake at five-something a.m. and I smiled at the first happy thought I'd had in days. My mother must have found a telephone in that jungle she was traipsing through and forgotten about time differences.

"Hello? Mom?" I answered eagerly.

"Lena? Sorry, no, this is Jarrod. Look, sorry to bother you at this hour, and on Christmas Day, too, but Barkley's top colt just tried to geld himself. I know you're not on call, but can you please come help me? I need you to do the anesthesia."

I let out my breath with a whoosh and swallowed the disappointment. The horse needed help and Jarrod was one of the practice partners.

No time for wobblies.

"Is he stable?" I heard myself ask.

"Seems to be."

"What's his color like, and is he bleeding?"

"His color is okay and he's only cut the scrotum, so there's not much blood, but I need you."

Barkley is our practice's top racing trainer and his horses were no slouches. "No" simply wasn't an option. Besides, if I couldn't spend Christmas with the people I loved, it might as well be with a horse.

They were always good for a cuddle.

Equally as important, unflappable Jarrod sounded downright shook.

"Of course, Boss, I'll be there. He's at the stable?"

"Yep. Thanks mate, I owe you." The relief in his voice was palpable.

"Not at all. Be right there."

I flew into my clothes and roared out the driveway only minutes later. Jarrod rarely asked for help and was generally bullet proof, certainly not a man to panic needlessly. I'd jumped into pens of rutting stags beside him to clip and TB test them—him because he was fearless and me because I had no idea how stupid it was and blindly followed him—wearing shorts, for Pete's sake.

Ten minutes later, I hopped out of my ute and trotted, stethoscope in hand, toward the barn, slowing my pace as I neared the crowd at the other end of the aisle. The stablemen opened a path to reveal the massive colt in all his shining splendor.

I blinked. And blinked again, but nothing changed as I

stared in horror. The right testicle of the top-selling colt at last year's Manukau Magic Billions sale hung free of the shredded remains of his scrotum, somewhere between the fidgeting bay's hocks.

I'm sure everyone heard my gulp. This wasn't a surgery we wanted to mess up. I'd watched this colt at the track and I had to agree he was unparalleled in this district, maybe even in all of New Zealand. The colt had been purchased for an exorbitant sum and was truly the prize of Barkleys' stable—not to mention the top breeding prospect of his syndicated owners.

The big, lanky bay kicked with annoyance at his naked nut. The pain must have been mind-bending. I took one look at Jarrod and headed back to my ute with the vet in hot pursuit. I began pulling out trays and filling them with catheters, flush, IV lines, anesthetic drugs, and fluid bags.

"I put a weight tape on him: 575 kilograms," Jarrod said, "and his lungs, trachea, heart rate and rhythm are fine." Jarrod sounded confident, but today, for the first time in my experience, he was pale beneath his tan.

"Great, thanks. No problem with anesthetics before?"

"None that Barkley knows about. And he was vaccinated for tetanus a few months ago. Otherwise healthy."

"Great, thanks. How'd he do it?"

"Went over the divider in the horse truck on the way home from the track."

"They're keen, working the horses on Christmas Day."

"I gather the horses get Boxing Day off, instead."

"Frank," I called to one of the hovering stablemen,

"could you please get me a couple buckets of hot water for these fluids?"

"No problem, be right there." He scuttled off.

"There's no way the colt can keep that dropped testicle," Jarrod said, "the remnants of the cremaster muscle have rubber-banded up inside him. Let's just geld him."

I nearly dropped my tray of already-filled syringes and struggled to draw a breath. "Are you out of your ever-lovin' mind?" I hissed from between gritted teeth and glanced at the faces of the assembled crowd in the barn looking curiously at us.

"He could get orchitis from having the scrotum ripped up and castrating only the right side."

"That's a chance I'm willing to take." I could breathe again, but my heart was still pounding. "Anti-inflammatories and antibiotics will help with that. We can always take the other testicle out later if it becomes a problem. The exposed one's been out for awhile and it's probably got to go, but he needs to keep that other one."

"I'm not so sure." Jarrod frowned.

"Look, do you want to keep your license to practice? That horse is worth more as a breeding prospect than the two of us put together." I stopped, staring and breathing hard. "Do you want to be the one to tell the syndicate bosses you removed his only remaining testicle on the *possibility* it could cause a problem? Do you know who they are? I do, and I have no desire to come to their attention in any sort of negative way. Horse heads in beds and all that. *No*." I shook my head. "*Just no*."

"I'll get my gear out," he whispered, and fled.

Mr. Barkley walked up, probably more pale than Jarrod, if that were possible.

"Sir," I said, and returned to my bottles, averting my eyes. He hadn't been keen on having me, a girl vet, on his farm before, but he wasn't prepared to argue right about now.

"Thank you for coming," he said softly, and met my gaze for a moment. I figured this was as close to an apology as I'd ever get.

"No problem," I said, and attempted a smile, but I fear it was more of a grimace.

"You know who this colt is?"

I nodded. "We'll do our best for him."

And we did. After I injected the anesthetic drugs into his catheter, he went down like a baby with my hands supporting both sides of his halter and lay still while I tied up his leg. Jarrod emasculated the loose testicle and cleaned up the area, then we left it open to drain.

"His left testicle is still fully enclosed," Jared murmured to me, "so I'm done here."

"Good job," I said, as I reached forward to tug the slip bowline from the rope holding his near hind up to his shoulder, then checked the padding between his head and the halter rings. I left the towel draped loosely over his top eye while he slept off the anesthetic drugs so he'd awaken gradually.

He sat up onto his chest ten minutes later, his head still wobbly, then climbed to his feet with my hands on his halter to stabilize his head.

Mr. Barkley stared. "I've never seen such a smooth recovery," he said, with a shake of his head.

"New drugs from the young girl vet," I couldn't help saying. My mother always told me it wasn't nice to smirk, so I bit my lips together instead and turned to watch the colt, who dropped his head to nose at the grass before him. He lipped at it ineffectively in his woozy state, but he was recovering well.

I gave him his antibiotics and anti-inflammatories via his catheter, then removed it when he was more awake. With a few strokes for the colt, I returned to my ute.

"The regular post-castration exercise?" Mr. Barkley called after me.

"Yes, give him 24 hours, then trot him ten minutes each way on the lunge twice a day. And for goodness sake, do *not* run water on it. Below the wound is fine." I'd seen people hose castration incisions too many times for my liking—it introduced bacteria that just didn't need to be in a clean wound.

He frowned, but nodded. "Thanks for coming, Lena. Sorry to interrupt your Christmas."

"It's fine. Not much on, anyway." Tears brimmed at his mention of the holiday. I turned away before they spilled out.

"Luckily we got you this morning," Jarrod said, then looked sideways at me. "Weren't you going away with your—"

"Was," I interrupted, swallowing hard, and swiped at the tears surreptitiously.

"Why don't you come around this afternoon? The family'd love to have you with us."

I gulped. "I'd like that, thanks." I packed up and even managed a smile as I waved and drove away.

Mr. Barkley flagged me down as I passed his house.

"Thank you—and Merry Christmas," he said. "There's something on your passenger seat. Don't drink it all at once."

I glanced across my cab to see a bottle of Courvoisier VSOP, complete with a glittering gold bow.

Merry Christmas, indeed.

It seemed I was on my way to acceptance—at work, anyway.

A CHRISTMAS AFTERNOON chocker-full of Jarrod and Janet's three young children and the rest of their relatives distracted me from my cares. They were all kind and impressed with Jarrod's and my exciting morning.

Janet was amazing. I'd marveled before at her skill of somehow remaining clean while working in her garden for hours at a time in classy, white clothing with her three small helpers upon my last visit. She did the same with a full Christmas dinner today. I have no idea how. I can't stay clean on a good day, even without children.

With a cheery wave I headed for home, my heart lighter than it'd been in days. As I stepped in the door, the piney scent of Christmas made my heart twinge. The only things missing were cinnamon and cloves—and my loved ones. I dropped to my knees before my little pine Christmas tree and sat still for a moment, just remembering.

One after the other, I touched the few precious ornaments I'd brought to New Zealand from California—one for every year, each encircled with its own memories. I held myself in check and tried to enjoy the memories, but as I turned on the string of lights at the wall, the tiny fairy lights blazed and I promptly had a meltdown.

I spent the next two hours trying to stop crying and draw myself out of this funk, all the while staring longingly at the glittering Courvoisier. I daren't start on it in this state.

A roll of wrapping paper, red on one side and white on the other, caught my eye and reminded me of the Danish Christmas tree baskets and snowflakes I made with my mum and sister so many years ago. I collected some scissors from the non-sterile spares kit in my vet truck and proceeded to make snowflakes. Many, many snowflakes. Big ones, little ones, and everything in between. I scattered some under the tree and taped others to the windows and gazed at them in the deepening twilight.

At an inspiration, I untaped the biggest ones and stood at the window, pencil in hand.

What did the holiday mean to me?

Christmas isn't about the presents or the getting.

I sat at the table and wrote in tiny letters—all around the edges of one snowflake—and then another.

It's about the giving of love, of caring to the people who love you and those you love—and sharing time with those most special to you.

I stopped and cried some more.

Giving of my time, my caring, to animals, people, and the earth.

And more.

The names of people who love me, those I love.

Eventually, I ran out of room to write, though the tears seemed limitless. The snowflakes were full, their writing in full circles—and I'd gone full circle along with them.

I sat gazing at the delicate snowflakes with their intricate cuts bordered by tiny lettering around the perimeters. I slowly pivoted them, reading around and around, thoughts repeated like a mantra. Repeated in hope the expressions of plenty would overpower my overwhelming sense of loss. It worked until I collapsed into a heap of tears.

Again.

But was everything really *that* bad? I had everything I could want—the fantastic new career I'd spent the past decade studying to obtain, a job in a great practice, and a wonderful new country of my own choosing. I should be satisfied—but I wasn't.

I gripped the biggest snowflake in my fingers, but it blurred before my eyes. Bed was probably the best place for me, though it wasn't even close to dark.

With one more glance at the little tree, I locked the doors. I thought the tree might cry as well—bereft of anything but the few presents I'd bought for others and not yet delivered—and a scattering of my snowflakes.

I picked up a handful of snowflakes from beneath a pine bough and took them to bed with me, focusing on the messages of love and care. My family seemed very far away tonight. If only—Nigel—but no, no use wishing for things I couldn't have. Christmas wasn't just about wishes. It just wasn't.

I tried to forget the joy of the past two months, but the days rolled over and over through my head as I lay awake, snowflakes clutched wetly to my chest.

I must have slept, if fitfully. Images of Nigel's stricken face, an upside down car, death, and destruction swirling through my dreams until a swirled beside the bed ripped me from my nightmares.

11

I leapt up in a panic until I realized it was the phone. In my haste to stop the demonic shriek, I knocked it off the table and had to dive down beside the bed to find it—nearly falling off in the process.

"Hello?" I asked, as civilly as possible through gritted teeth.

"Lena, can ye come?" The strain in the elderly gentleman's voice cooled my temper in a way ice could never do. A familiar voice… but whose?

"Lena? It's D—" the man's voice cut out.

"Don, is that you?"

"Yes, lass, it's m—"

The phone line was terrible, but I'd never heard him sound this worried.

Oh my God, no. I broke out into a cold sweat. *Ben.* It could only be Ben—*or Nigel*. My eyes snapped fully open and my head cleared.

"Of course," I said, as I swung my legs out of bed and rubbed my streaming eyes. "Just a mo."

"Sorry to bother—this early—out mov—stock…" The line crackled, then was silent.

I gulped and glanced at the clock. Nearly 10 p.m., and nearly dark.

"Is it Ben?"

"How's that?"

"Is it Ben?" I shouted into the phone.

"—not so good today."

After fifteen years chasing sheep and cattle on Don's steep cliffs, tongue lolling, his lips pulled back into a grin, I thought he'd done pretty well, myself. Most working sheep dogs here didn't live half that long.

"Down the back—farm—reception—left the old boy in —house. Howling the place—he was, had to—him home, he hates…" his voice trailed off.

I shuddered. *Down the back of the farm.* I didn't think there *was* any cell phone coverage out there at all. I quivered, guts tensing at the thought of the special afternoon I'd spent with Nigel out there, and dragged my thoughts back to where they belonged.

"On my way."

"See you—house," he said.

Other than an incredible blanket of stars covering the dark sky, only a few lights showed across the countryside at this hour. The tiny sparks of farm bikes bounced their way across paddocks to finish putting the dairy cows away after a late Christmas milking and clumps of dazzling brilliance marked the remote milking sheds. I always thought they reminded me of something out of *Dune*—the sudden blaze looking like a factory in the middle of the sands of nowhere.

My mind drifted into that half-alert state in which country veterinarians seem to survive.

Farm bikes drew my memories back to Nigel and Don's farm. Though it was only a few weeks it felt like forever ago —and my heart wrenched.

Leave it, said the little voice on my shoulder. *You have other things to worry about tonight.*

I flew past the faded once-were-townships of Pokuru and Te Kawa and somehow the ute stuck to the winding roads. The lights of Otorohanga blazed for a few minutes, before they, too, were gone from my rearview mirror. Right at the deathtrap of a Waitomo turnoff, then past the signs for the limestone caves and Waitomo Caves Hotel.

The two-lane country road narrowed even further as the vet truck and I negotiated the tortuous bends between Waitomo and the coast. Rounding a corner in a dense stand of bush, my headlights picked out a flash of white fur in the middle of the one-lane road before me.

Hell.

I slammed on the brakes. Somehow, the ute juddered to a halt on the hairpin turn just before I hit it.

Heart in my mouth, praying someone hadn't smacked it with a car already, I leapt from the cab. The tiny black and white pup cowered just in front of my wheel.

He was shaking, heck, *I* was shaking. When he saw me in the headlights, he started to whine and came to me. I carefully scooped him up and gave him a once-over in the patch of bright moonlight beside the door. I could finally let out the breath I'd been holding. He was alive and well. Something was right in the world tonight—this pup was needed.

I slipped the little guy into the copious pocket of my outback jacket and slid back into the cab, grateful to my mechanic and the universe for the little life warming my hip.

With half an hour more traveling to go, I settled back down to drive.

Nigel.

I had time to think now and my mind was finally clear. What could I do to get over this? The man would clearly never believe me, probably would never believe anyone. Who was I to think I could make a difference?

When—if—he returned to town, perhaps we could speak. More likely, he'd see me in the street and turn the other way. My guts flipped over.

Maybe thinking about this wasn't such a good idea. Instead, I cupped the little sleeping life in my pocket between downshifting for the tight bends in the road.

I shot through Te Anga, then turned left at the Marokopa turnoff, flying along the long straight stretches until I reached Marokopa, then a hard left up the hill towards my final destination, doing everything in my power to think of *anything* other than Nigel.

I shook myself at the sight of Don's gateway and skidded to a halt. Grabbing my emergency bag, I hurried out of the car, barely noticing the other ute parked beside Don's Land Cruiser.

I forgot all about Nigel until he appeared in front of me

like a wraith. I shook my head to clear it of the apparition, but it still stood there, blocking the gateway.

"Leave me alone," I said, with a shudder, and made to walk through the vision, but Nigel was very real. His chest where I rammed into him was solid hard, warm flesh. I leapt back, wringing my hands where I'd touched him.

"What the hell are you doing here?" he growled.

"I might ask you the same thing," I said. "Don rang—"

"Lena," Don called, as he trotted down the steps toward me. "Oh, Nigel, there you are. Lena, come on in." Don grabbed my hand and tugged me up the stairs and through the house, tears streaming from his reddened eyes.

"Thank you for coming," Don said, then wiped his sleeve across his eyes. "Ben wasn't good when I left him this evening to check on a heifer down the farm. That's why I called you. I'm sorry to disturb your Christmas."

Don closed his eyes inhaled deeply, then bit his lips together for a moment. "I just got home. Ben waited for me, Lena… he licked my hand, closed his eyes, then was… *gone*." The last at a whisper.

The dog's grizzled head lay on Don's pillow, eyes closed.

"Poor old man," I said, stroking his soft fur. "But how many working dogs get to end their days on their favorite people's pillow?"

"Thank you so much for coming, Lena," Don said, then broke down beside Ben, sobbing as if his heart would break. I put an arm around him, but I don't think he even knew I was there.

I glanced up to see Nigel holding up the doorway, his face unreadable and his body rigid.

Don slowly quieted and I reached into my pocket. The little beggar had gone to sleep. I lifted him out carefully and slid him beneath Don's armpit. The pup awakened, whined, and squirmed until he came up for air beside the old man's face.

"What the?" Don slowly straightened up, staring at the tiny sheepdog pup. He looked up at me curiously, shivered, then curled himself around both the wee dog and his old friend, crooning softly to them both.

"He was nearly road pizza," I whispered, "but I guess Ben knew you needed help, so here he is." I straightened and stepped backwards toward the door, watching the three figures on the bed.

I only remembered Nigel was there when I backed straight into him.

12

"Oof"—I jumped when my body contacted Nigel's in the doorway and lost my balance, but his arms around me kept me from landing on the floor—"What are you doi—"

"Ssh," Nigel cut off my furious whisper with one of his own and he nodded at Don on the bed.

We both stepped backward and out the door, and I glanced back at Don in time to see him look at us with the first smile I'd seen since I arrived.

Out in the hallway, Nigel dropped his arms away from me and closed the door in front of me as I turned to leave.

"Where do you think you're going and why are you here?"

"Isn't that fairly obvious?" I growled as my heart pounded in my chest. "Your uncle rang and asked me to come."

"Why?"

"He was worried about Ben. What the hell are you doing out here? Your mother's worried sick."

"Hiding out."

"*Really?*" His flip response sparked my anger and I wanted… I'm not sure what, but at least I wanted a decent response from him. I'd spent so much of myself worrying about him for weeks, and this was the best he could do? "Isn't it time you grew up and got over yourself?"

"What do you know about it?" he hissed.

"Enough to see what's in front of my eyes," I snapped.

"And what's that?" he said, barely audible, but I heard him because he was only a breath away from me, his arms on either side of me against the wall.

"That you're afraid to try again," I spat. "That you want love and are capable of giving love, but you're not willing to even *try*."

He closed his eyes for a moment, his jaw tensed. "So tell me the truth about Madsen."

"What truth about Madsen? That we had one disastrous date and I walked two miles home barefoot rather than get in the car with him again? You've got it *so* wrong. I have no idea why I've been pining for you since you ran away from the saleyards."

His eyes jerked up to mine. "You've been… ran away?" He didn't seem to know which part of our conversation to focus upon.

"Yes, ran away. You wouldn't even talk with me."

"But you were—"

"*Waiting for you.* I was *waiting for you.*"

"But Madsen—"

"He appeared out of nowhere, just as you showed up. So help me God."

He froze and his arms dropped to his sides.

"I couldn't—I couldn't be responsible for—"

"And you *wouldn't*. You weren't responsible for your wife's death, not directly."

He stiffened and I thought he was going to bolt again, so I grabbed his shirt front and held on for dear life.

"You *know?*"

I nodded and leaned my forehead on his chest. Wishing, begging, inside my head. Afraid to speak. Afraid I'd never see him again.

He didn't say a word for long minutes. Finally he spoke. "Did you mean that?"

"What?" I breathed, afraid to trust my voice.

"About missing me."

I lifted my head and our eyes locked. "Of course, you great lug. I've missed you every minute of every day. Christmas has been a nightmare—in more ways than one."

"Not half as much as I've missed you." He wrapped his arms around me and held me. Held me as I'd dreamed he would, for these long weeks—and then his mouth was on mine. The minutes stretched out to infinity as our hunger for each other blanked out the rest of the world.

I don't know how long we'd have stood in the hallway in each other's arms if Don hadn't come out of his room with the pup, tears still in his eyes, but purpose in his gait.

"About time you two figured this out. Nigel, meet Lena. Lena, Nigel. I see you've kissed and made up, now get on the phone and ring your poor mother, young man, and wish her a happy holiday. Then take yourselves off home. Merry Christmas to you both, thank you for coming out, Lena, and I hope you both got your Christmas wishes," he said, as he headed into the kitchen.

"Guess we've been told," Nigel said, and kissed me on the forehead. "Merry Christmas. Now I've got my wish."

My smile probably lit up the night.

"So have I, and with only," I glanced at my watch, "two minutes to spare. But seriously, Nigel, do you finally believe me?"

He took a deep breath and looked me in the eyes, his own finally clear. I could see all the way into his soul for the very first time.

"Yes, I do. Are you willing to let me try again… to love you properly this time, no shadows?"

"Lead the way, Nigel, lead the way," I said, as our lips met once again.

EPILOGUE

The sun glistened off the sea as the whole Munro family, plus one, relaxed in the warm black sand beside the river mouth at Marokopa Beach.

I reached out for Nigel's hand and he turned his head to gaze up at me with a lazy smile.

"We didn't make it out here for Christmas, but we couldn't miss New Year's," Sara said, her gaze locking with mine.

"So glad we could come out. I wouldn't have missed this for the world."

"Oh," John said, "I nearly forgot. Lena, you're safe to eat ice cream again."

"Pardon?"

"Well, remember that cowshed next door to us where the two of you met?"

I shuddered as I met Nigel's eyes. "I'm afraid I can't forget that one."

"Well," John continued, "the dairy company's been

visiting. I don't think they'll be putting a cow through that shed for quite some time, if ever. I believe he's buying the shed next door to him for the time being. And improving sanitation."

"Well, that's a relief," I said, finally letting my breath out.

"And now we can eat our dessert," Sara said, reaching for the chilly bin. "Homemade chocolate ice cream!"

Thank you for joining Lena in
Greener Pastures Calling.
Lena will be returning in other books in the series.

Enjoyed the story? Want to read more?
If you loved it, a short review on Bookbub, Goodreads and your favorite eBook retailer would sure be appreciated.
I'd be grateful for your help in spreading the word!

Sign up for Lizzi's VIP Reader Club to hear about new releases and specials, plus get your free sampler gift at
www.lizzitremayne/VIPGREEN

FIND BOOKS

Find eBooks at your favorite online retailer via buy links at www.lizzitremayne.com

or

Purchase Softcover books:

from New Zealand and Australia,

My print books are available in standard (and some in large format) print for your reading pleasure. Find bookstores stocking my books at:

www.lizzitremayne.com/Booksellers

From Other Countries:

Print books are available in paperback from most online retailers and in select bookstores around the world.

Find stockists at www.lizzitremayne.com/Booksellers

BOOKS BY THE AUTHOR

The Long Trails Series

Books 1-3: ***The Long Trails Box Set: Historical Western Family Saga: Books 1-3***

Can an orphan, with only her Mustang and a Cossack sword, survive alone on the frontier?

From the deserts of Utah, through the gold mines of California, to the turbulent wilderness of Colonial New Zealand, Aleksandra rides, loves, and fights—with only her Cossack skills to keep her alive.

Book One: ***A Long Trail Rolling***

Hunted for her secrets. Hiding in plain sight. Can one woman blaze her own trail into untamed territory?

Winner of the True West Magazine 2016 Best Western Romance, Winner Romance Writers of New Zealand: 2014 Pacific Hearts Award and 2015 Koru Award

UTAH TERRITORY, 1860. Aleksandra has spent her whole life training for the inevitable. So, when a brutal Cossack tracks down and kills her father, she instinctively collects her pa's elixir and flees. But when she meets the mysterious Xavier at a nearby trading post, she wonders if she can win both his protection and his heart…

Disappointed when the man of her dreams leaves to join the Pony Express, Aleksandra dons a disguise to follow him into the dangerous frontier assignment. Hiding behind her martial arts skills and a male alias, she longs to tell the handsome Xavier the truth. But with the killer in pursuit, keeping up the ruse may be her only chance for survival...

Can Aleksandra save both her love and her family legacy from a relentless murderer?

Book Two: ***The Hills of Gold Unchanging***

As the Civil War rages, secessionists menace California. The Confederates want the state and they'll stop at nothing to take it.

UTAH TERRITORY, 1860. On a wagon train headed West, Aleksandra makes an enemy of a gun-running Confederate when she fights her way out of his unwelcome embrace and Xavier's new friends realize he's heard too much to be allowed to live. Embroiled in the Confederate's fight to drag the new state from the Union and make it their own, can Aleks and Xavier survive? The secessionists mean business.

Book Three: ***A Sea of Green Unfolding***

They set sail for the peace and calm of New Zealand, but they hadn't counted on murderers, mutineers, and a land war in paradise.

SAN FRANCISCO BAY AND NEW ZEALAND, 1863. Tragedy strikes in Aleksandra and Xavier's newly found paradise on their California Rancho but Von Tempsky's invitation draws them to a new life in peaceful New Zealand. They disembark into a turbulent wilderness—with the opening shots of the New Zealand Wars just being fired—straight at them.

Novella: **Somewhere Called Home**

Highlands to Waterloo—can love prevail over fate?

SCOTTISH HIGHLANDS, 1813.

Robert is disowned for refusing to become clan tacksman after his father and heads for the city, alone, to build a life for himself and his beloved Sofia. Sofia's waiting turns to despair when her mother buys safety during the clearance of their village—leaving Sofia at the mercy of the laird's degenerate son. Rob emerges from the hell of Waterloo wanting only to see Sofia again... and his father. *To be released soon.*

The *Tatiana* Series

(with links to The Long Trails series)

Book One: **Tatiana I**

Stableman's daughter Tatiana rises to glamorous heights by her equestrienne abilities—but the tsar's glittering attention is not always gold.

MOSKVA, RUSSIA 1842. Tatiana and her husband Vladimir become pawns in the emperor's pursuit of a coveted secret weapon. While Tatiana and their infant son are placed under house arrest, Vladimir must recover the weapon or lose his wife and young son. With the odds mounting against them, can they find each other again—half a world away? *Coming soon!*

The Once Upon a Vet School Series

Drama and humor abound as Lena pursues her childhood

dream of becoming an equine vet—and beyond—in this unique series of

six independent novella sequences:

~Junior Years~

After Lena hears she needs good grades to become a veterinarian, things start to get tricky. Even her pony doesn't get out unscathed. (Middle Grade) ***USA 1972-1976***

~High School Days ~

When your high school counsellor says vet school's too hard for you and your HS sweetheart offers you a dream life of farming, writing, and babies, what do you do? Is vet school really the be-all, end-all? (Young Adult) ***USA 1976-1979***

~College Nights~

How can you have a life when you need an A in every class for four years to get into vet school... on top of 800 hours vet practice work? Something's got to give. (Young Adult and up) ***USA 1980-1984***

~Vet School 24/7~

Now they're in, the pressure for grades is off and vet school social life is upon them... there's only the tsunami of 200 years of veterinary knowledge to pack into their heads. Can Lena and her friends stay afloat? (Young Adult and up) ***USA 1984-1988***

~Practice Time~

Finally graduated, prima ballerinas of the university, Lena and her vet school classmates disperse to far-flung practices... and real life.

What could possibly go wrong? Late nights on-call, mud, blood, and finally, a light at the end of the tunnel... unfortunately, it's only the penlight of a dictatorial vet technician in Lena's eyes after she passed out on the floor. (Women's Rural Fiction with Romantic Elements) ***USA & New Zealand 1988-2012***

~Long in the Tooth~

When Lena suffers another catastrophic back injury in New Zealand, what's she to do to feed her family and keep the farm? She can't breathe around cats or birds and what good's an equine vet who can't hold up a horse's leg? Time for Lena to go back to school. Again. (Women's Rural Fiction with Romantic Elements) ***New Zealand 2012- ...***

Currently Available Reads:

~Vet School 24/7~

Fifty Miles at a Breath

Horses bring them together and their future looks rosy—it's the present they can't handle.

When equine veterinary student Lena and veteran pilot Blake fall in love, vet school and the past intrude. Add in a long-distance relationship, and things get just plain hard. A grueling endurance race forces them to draw on their strengths and face their fears —together.

Lena Takes a Foal

She needs help... he needs to stay away...

Lena's got a problem—one that might prevent her from graduating. When her horse flips over and lands on her, it has to be the dashing resident, Kit, who finds her. Luckily, she's sworn off relationships after her last debacle and sea-green eyes and rugged good looks are the last things on her mind. Besides, to a veterinary school faculty, relationships between residents and students are like oil and water.

They just don't mix.

~Practice Time~

Greener Pastures Calling

A new country, a great job, and a good Kiwi bloke. Life couldn't be better.

Until it gets worse.

Newly emigrated to New Zealand, Lena wants a 'good Kiwi bloke', but they're elusive as their nocturnal namesake. Nigel's avoiding females, unless they're cows, horses, or his mother after his first marriage. Sparks fly when they meet—but not the first time, over the dirty instruments in a filthy cowshed. They seem to be made for each other, until Nigel remembers where he first saw her. And then the questions start.

Understanding Modern Vet Med for Owners

The new series of veterinary books for horse owners to let you use what vets know to keep your horses healthier and happier. *First volume due out soon!*

With Bluestocking Belles

Boxed sets of historical love stories from a host of bestselling authors.

Christmas 2018: *Follow Your Star Home*

The Viking star ring is said to bring lovers together, no matter how far, no matter how hard.

In nine stories, covering more than half the world and a thousand years, our heroes and heroines put the legend to the test. Watch the star work its magic, as prodigals return home in the season of good will, uncertain of their welcome.

With Authors of Main Street

Boxed sets of *new* contemporary love stories from multiple bestselling authors, for a sweet romantic holiday treat.

Christmas 2017: *Christmas Babies on Main Street Nine stories from the bestselling Authors of Main Street!*

From the small hamlet of Eastport, to the gorgeous landscapes of New Zealand, to Main Street, USA, you'll find the Christmas spirit and warm love stories on every page.

Summer 2018: *Summer Romance on Main Street*

Seven stories from the Authors of Main Street!

Welcome to Main Street, where you'll find sweet summer romance and true love from small towns everywhere

Christmas 2018: *Christmas Wishes on Main Street*

Seven stories from the Authors of Main Street

Don't you love to hear everyone's Christmas wishes? Read our small town wishes and feel the love from Canada all the way through to New Zealand.

Sign up for Lizzi's VIP Reader Club to hear about new releases and specials, plus get your free sampler gift here!

www.lizzitremayne.com/VIPLong

Lizzi Tremayne's Books
2019

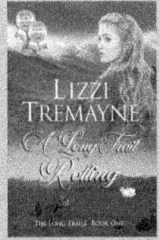
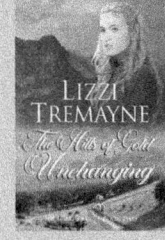
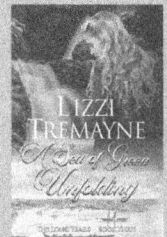

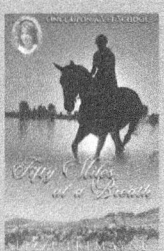
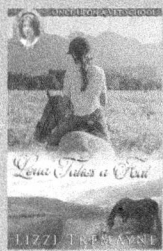
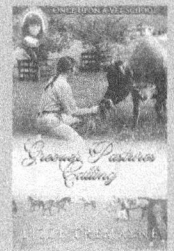

Coming Soon!

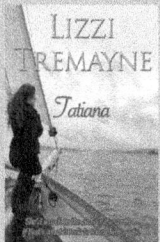
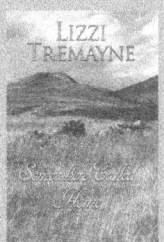

With Love From
New Zealand, Russia, Scotland, and U.S.A.

AUTHOR'S NOTES

On the off chance that you haven't figured it out by now, much of this series is based upon my life and times before, during, and after veterinary school. Some is fictitious and some is not, in answer to some of my readers' questions.

My favorite book as a young pre-teen was Mary Stewart's *Airs Above the Ground*. I have always loved history, travel, veterinary medicine, and horses (especially Lippizaners), but not necessarily in that order. Ms. Stewart's book had it all. My love for this combination was one of my main reasons for writing the *Once Upon a Vet School* series. I read *Airs Above the Ground* so many times, the cover and first two pages are detached... but I still have them. Yep, after all these years. My only regret was that I never met the author. She died just before I began writing... around the time I learned one could actually contact authors.

Dreams can indeed come true. Becoming a veterinarian was

my dream from the age of seven. If this is your dream, never, *ever* let anyone dissuade you. Don't listen to well-meaning high school counselors when they attempt to offer you 'easier' choices. It almost deterred me, but thanks to Dr. Karsten Fostvedt and his then-wife Susan, I got back on my horse. The rest is history.

I hope you enjoy your foray into my world of veterinary fiction. If you liked it, help others find it by leaving reviews and comments where you purchased it, on Bookbub, Goodreads, and on my webpage. If you want to pass on a comment, please find me via my *Connect with Lizzi* page.

Warmest regards,

Lizzi Tremayne

RECIPE: WHITEBAIT FRITTERS

Whisk in bowl until light and frothy:

- 2 eggs

Add and mix well:

- 1 c (250 g) whitebait
- 1 pinch sea salt flakes
- ground white or black pepper to taste

Heat together over medium heat in large heavy frying pan:

- 2 Tbs (30 ml) Oil
- 2 Tbs (30 ml) Butter

When butter starts to bubble and spit, spoon tablespoons of the egg/whitebait mixture into the pan. Can cook 5-6 of them at a time, depending upon the size of your pan.

Fry for a minute or two, then turn once to cook other side.

Do not overcook, they're delicate!

Serve immediately (or place onto warmed plate) and keep cooking until they're all fried.

Serve with:
lemon wedges!

Bon appétit!

ABOUT THE AUTHOR

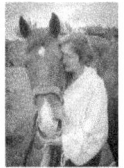

Lizzi grew up riding wild in the Santa Cruz Mountain redwoods, became an equine veterinarian at UC Davis School of Veterinary Medicine and practiced in the Gold and Pony Express Country of California before emigrating to New Zealand. She has two wonderful boys, a grandbaby, and an awesome partner in that sea of green. When she's not writing, she's swinging a rapier or shooting a bow in medieval garb, riding or driving a carriage, playing in the garden on her hobby farm, singing, cooking, or looking into a horse's mouth in her equine veterinary dental practice. She is multiply published and awarded in special interest magazines and veterinary periodicals.

With this debut novel, she was Finalist 2013 RWNZ Great Beginnings, Winner 2014 RWNZ Pacific Hearts Award for the unpublished full manuscript, Winner 2015 RWNZ Koru Award for Best First Novel and third in Koru Long Novel, and Finalist 2015 Best Indie Book Award.

CONNECT WITH LIZZI

I'm looking forward to hearing from you!

Join conversations and find story excerpts, buy links, and more here:

www.lizzitremayne.com/VIPGREEN
www.lizzitremayne.com
www.horseandvetbooks.com
www.bookandmainbites.com/LizziTremayne/
www.bookbub.com/profile/lizzi-tremayne/
www.facebook.com/lizzitremayneauthor/
www.instagram.com/lizzitremayne/
www.twitter.com/LizziTremayne/
www.youtube.com/user/lizzikiwi/
www.goodreads.com/LizziTremayne/
https://nz.pinterest.com/lizzitremayne/

ACKNOWLEDGEMENTS

~A huge appreciation for my wonderful friends and beta readers, who, incidentally, did this on ridiculously short notice… dare I say once again? Thank you to Elizabeth Ellen Carter, Kirsten Davidson, Matthew Tremayne, Rue Allyn, and Jude Knight. Thank you Marjorie Cooke, who edited this for the anthology with the Authors of Main Street, and to the other Authors of Main Street. You're a great bunch of gals! Your consideration and wonderful ideas improved this story.

~Thank you to Meredith Reece for helping me choose the title for this story. You suggested *Greener Pastures*. I can't seem to manage short titles, and there were far too many books with that title, so I added *Calling*. As a fellow author, you'll understand why!

~Thank you to mum, who found the ONE cover image we ransacked two houses to find. Good job. The cover is immensely better for the lovely photo you took all those years ago.

~Thank you to all the dairy great veterinarians with whom I worked with when I first came to New Zealand—John Harrison, Mike Woods, Brian McKay, Steve Murray, Noel Powers, Richard Jerram, and Neil Houston… and our indomitable office manager, Kathy, who kept us all on our toes.

~And last, but not least, my gratitude also goes to the veterinarians who either collaborated with me, encouraged me to speak and publish on complimentary therapies, or referred their valued clients and patients for Postural Rehabilitation back in the early days when there were exceedingly few people, and no veterinarians, doing bodywork on New Zealand horses. Thank you for helping so many horses—David Sim, Corin Murfitt, Mark Ethell, Ian Robertson, Nigel Perkins, and many others.

Thank you all!

xx

Lizzi

EXCERPT FROM A LONG TRAIL ROLLING

A *pril 1860, Echo Canyon, Utah Territory, U.S.A.*

SHE SMELLED BLOOD. Its metallic tang assailed her senses before it was overshadowed by the stench of death. Stepping back to scan the sheer wall of the bluff rising before her, her breath caught in her throat and a sob escaped.

Finally, she'd found him.

A scuffed black boot and fur coat showed through the snow, his body wedged into the bottom of a crevice three feet above her head. She looked up to the top of the cliff, from which he must have fallen, but saw no one.

Finding handholds where there were none, Aleksandra Lekarski scrambled up the wall as her heart constricted in her chest. She tugged her father's cold, stiff body free and down onto level ground, giving thanks he'd been out of reach of the wolves whose tracks abounded in the snow where she now stood. Her world blurred as she dropped to her knees and cradled his lifeless head in her lap, rocking him. Ceaseless tears flowed down her doeskin tunic.

With a numbing pain in her mind, she ran shaking hands over him, seeking answers. What could have made an experienced trapper like Krzysztof Lekarski fall off a bluff and succumb to a death more suited to a greenhorn?

This couldn't really be happening.

Just seven days ago, he'd kissed her goodbye with glowing eyes.

'Keep the fire going in the smokehouse this time, will you, Aleks?'

'Of course, Papa, my promise. Be back soon, I'll miss you.'

'I'll return before you've missed me, then we'll go sell last winter's furs at the trading post.'

We'll never go to town together again.

Aleksandra sat back on her heels and gripped her swimming head in her hands, fingers pulling her hair until it hurt, then whimpered and returned her attention to her papa.

She shrank from what was left of his eyes… and was glad he'd been in the narrow gap, too small for large predators. Beetles had been there, or some rodent, maybe even a hawk. The scent of decay was a sharp contrast to the clean bite of fresh snow. Trying not to breathe through her nose, she swallowed hard, stomach rolling.

Aleksandra's hands froze as hard-crusted blood met her fingertips. Her heart stopped altogether at the sight of the inch-long, bloodied cut in his buckskin jerkin, repeating into his chest wall. She turned him over. A laceration of the same size exited the soft leather covering his back.

Papa hadn't simply fallen off the bluff. Nothing but a sword made such a wound.

Aleksandra's ears began to ring, her world narrowing to a small gap, as she fought the rising panic.

It couldn't be…Vladimir couldn't *have found us. Not over two decades, two continents and the Atlantic Ocean.*

The ground swayed as she hunched over her father's still form. Squeezing her eyes shut to stop the motion, she recalled the words Papa had endlessly repeated, so she would always remember:

'He *will* seek us out. Vladimir will come for the secret and we must be prepared to keep it from him—at all costs —always.'

But what a cost.

Despite her entire being screaming to fall apart for the loss of her only remaining family, years of Papa's training to protect their secret stopped her in her tracks. Struggling to draw air into her lungs, she looked around the bottom of the cliff. Her clearing vision now showed more wolf sign: scrapings on the wall below his body and white snow darkened by blood beside stinking yellow patches.

Leaving his body here, knowing the scavengers would return, would be the hardest thing she'd ever done—but Aleksandra knew what her papa would have required of her.

Heart sinking, she slumped to the forest floor beside him and took a deep breath of the wind whistling cold up the valley. Closing her eyes, she touched her lips to the top of his head. With shaking hands and tears flowing anew,

Aleksandra lifted the leather thong of the beaded *Shoshone* medicine bag from about his neck and pulled the signet ring from his finger. Kissing her papa once more, she covered him with dead leaves and snow, beseeching the forest spirits to care for him with love, if she couldn't return.

She rose and turned to leave, but through the brain-fogging misery, she remembered to check for the tools of Papa's trade. The trapper's sword scabbard was empty and his rifle missing. The firearm was nearby, half covered by a snowy branch, but even after searching for precious minutes, his *shashka* was nowhere to be found. With a twinge of regret, she gave up seeking her father's Cossack sword. She shouldered the rifle and stared back at the man she loved beyond life, her heart in a vise, with a promise and a prayer for his soul. Tears dried cold and tight on her face as she stood gazing past the putrefying corpse to the heart of her papa. She returned once more to brush back the frozen leaves and kiss him goodbye.

Her eyes scanned the aspen glade in the brilliant morning light. No one watched. With the silence and speed of the *kwahaten*, the antelope, her name with the *Shoshone* people who had welcomed her family into their own, she ran for her pony.

'It's you and me now, Dzień,' she choked out as she untied him and slung the rifle on her back. Vaulting on as he struck off into a lope, they flew back toward the cabin, the Indian pony seeming to sense the urgency and single-mindedness of his mistress. Slowing him to a stealthy walk as they neared the cabin, she slid from Dzień's back, signaling him to wait. She crept closer to the cabin. Before its open door, papers lay scattered beneath a light dusting of snow, fluttering in the chill breeze. The open barn doors slowly swung back and forth.

By now Papa's stallion should have been tearing up the stable and his field, but Rogan was gone. She waited, straining every muscle for any sound, but only silence met her ears, save the creaking hinges. She tiptoed around the perimeter of the yard in soft deerskin moccasins, keeping to the tree shadows as she'd done with her *Shoshone* friends in play. Hidden in shadow, Aleksandra stole to the window at the back of the cabin and peered in.

Her breath caught at the destruction. An intruder had turned the cabin upside down and must have set-to the place with a sword. The white softness of sliced feather-tick mattresses covered every surface and bedclothes were ribboned and strewn over the floorboards, but there was no movement. She eased the door open and slid inside, hand on the hilt of her own *shashka*.

The doors of the oak secretary, Krzysztof's gift to Aleksandra's mother just before her death two winters ago, lay open. She nearly cried to see its drawers flung helter-skelter and papers scattered.

Utensils danced amongst broken crockery and cast iron pans. In some dim recess of her mind, she noticed the *zakwas* and sourdough pots still stood on their shelf behind the cook stove, high above the chaos.

She broke into a sweat at the sight of the stove lids lying in deep, black grooves in the wooden floor of the cabin. Lids hot enough to burn themselves into the cedar planks meant she'd narrowly missed the visit of the intruder when she left the cabin to find her pa.

She froze. Nothing of value seemed to be missing. This was only a search. Her heart sank further at the sight of the sun-bleached muslin dress on its peg in the corner by her bed, doubtless informing the unwelcome visitor, by now almost certainly the Russian Vladimir, that someone besides Krzysztof lived here.

Aleksandra climbed onto the table and peered up into the eaves. Papa's velvet-lined boxes were still in their places. She lifted the lids and nearly smiled, then hopped down and slipped out the door. Skirting the yard again, she noiselessly opened the back door of the barn and peeked in. The summer smell of new hay assailed her nostrils as she entered and surveyed the damage. The trespasser had been busy here too.

Harnesses and building tools were scattered about the dirt floor, the contents of the feed room and hay pile scattered.

Well, that accounts for the scent.

The buckboard wagon and dogcart were still there, but the gate rails of Rogan's loosebox lay where they'd been dropped. The manure in the stall was dry, several days old.

She glanced around the darkened corners of the barn and the yard outside once more before returning to squeeze her hand into the secret cache behind the colt's feed bin. As her fingers chilled at the touch of the dozen or so frigid glass vials and the box next to it, her lips twisted into a bittersweet smile. For the first time in days, the leaden melancholy lifted from her shoulders, if only a little.

Despite the destruction, Vladimir had missed what he came for.

What now? Aleksandra ruminated, shaking her head, then took a great lungful of air.

Dzień trotted up at her whistle and she resolutely wiped her tears onto his mane, then hugged him around the neck with the hint of a smile.

'Papa's secret is safe, Dzień. We can bring him home,' she murmured, pressing her face into his furry neck. Reaching around, he nuzzled her derriere in reply and Aleksandra twisted to kiss him on his white star. She pulled the bedroll and bags from her saddle, then led him to the travois just inside the barn. She adjusted the two long poles, bound together with woven rawhide strips, then covered the widest part of the litter with a buffalo rug. Her papa's conveyance was complete.

On the long walk back to the bluff, she thought of her father's loving touch, his constant presence in her life, his sweet smile, his twinkling eyes. She would have them no more. Spiraling downward again, the thought of drowning in the emptiness was almost welcome, but she gritted her teeth and mentally shook herself. The focus was now on survival. Aleksandra suspected Vladimir didn't know the exact nature of what he sought, but nonetheless, he would return. She needed to be ready. Better yet, gone.

Aleksandra didn't fool herself. Her father, a survivor of Austro-Hungarian-occupied Poland, spent countless hours teaching his children self-defense. Unfortunately, Aleksandra's skills with a *shashka* were a fraction of those of her papa's… and even less than those of *his* own teacher,

Vladimir. The Russian was, according to Papa, unsurpassed with the short Russian Cossack sword.

'You're a good swordsman, Aleks, but your impetuosity gets you into trouble,' Papa always said, shaking his head as he disarmed her, yet again. The last time, he'd added: '… whether you're sparring at *shashkas* or trying to knit for the memory of your mama, God rest her soul, who tried to reconcile you to your femaleness.'

Aleksandra grinned through her tears. Knitting that always ended up as a wad of uneven and dropped stitches—inevitably thrown in fit of temper onto a set of antlers high upon the sitting room wall.

ROUNDING the bottom of the bluff, Dzień picked up his head and pricked his ears, sniffing the breeze, then headed for the pile of leaves covering Krzysztof. He stopped dead six feet away.

Aleksandra gave him a pat on the neck and tried to smile, but failed. She left the pony's head to adjust the travois. Breathing deeply through flared nostrils, Dzień stepped towards Krzysztof. He shook his mane, then nuzzled the lifeless body, knocking off the leaves as he checked the man's full length. Dzień tapped him with a front hoof, then snorted and turned away, showing the whites of his eyes as he stared at the motionless man from the corner of one eye. Aleksandra's gut wrenched.

Blood pounded in her head as she struggled to drag Krzysztof's six-foot frame onto the makeshift stretcher.

Dzień craned his neck around to watch, his muzzle and the skin about his eyes tensed and strained.

The pony responded to Aleksandra's gentle urging and took Krzysztof home one last time. She would bury him with his beloved wife and sons in their overpopulated graveyard, then determine how to elude Vladimir and survive.

'Can't protect our secret if you're dead, *moje drogie córki.*' Papa's words came back to her, in his thickly accented but precise English.

"*My darling daughter.*" Gulping, she clutched her father's medicine bag and choked back more tears, realizing she'd never hear those words again.

Want to read on? www.lizzitremayne.com/books
Sign up for Lizzi's VIP Reader Club to hear about new releases and specials, plus get your free sampler gift at www.lizzitremayne/VIPGREEN

EXCERPT FROM TATIANA

M*id-1842 Moskva, Russia*

BY THE TIME I was fifteen, and Vladimir sixteen, we were inseparable. No longer did he clean stalls as punishment, but to help me before his Training School classes began. This gave us more time to fit ourselves and prepare our combined *džigitovka* performances. We had been selected as part of the team to perform for the Tsar on his next visit to Moskva from St. Petersburg.

The tsar's creepy messenger, who came to our door with increasing regularity for no seemingly good reason, had delivered the invitation for our group to give the performance. His terse smile showed through the lace curtains as he stood before the door. I managed to talk Papa into answering it, claiming I couldn't leave my cooking pot.

The messenger, whose name I never asked, but he told

me anyway, was Sambor Andropov. Due to his frequent visits, I had taken to ignoring anyone knocking on the door when I was in the house alone. His mere eyes on me made my skin crawl, and I felt I was being undressed before his eyes. Although a servant of the tsar could not be ignored without serious repercussion, if he didn't know I was there, all would be well. If the message was important, he would return, or Mrs. Bagrov would get the door if she was in.

I had the grace to be embarrassed when I realized he had carried such a special invitation to our door after I had avoided him. It was just that men and boys in Papa stableyard never looked at me like that, so perhaps I was being overly sensitive. I vowed to be kinder to him when I saw him next. He was, after all, just doing the tsar's bidding.

After this missive, our training intensified. We only had a month to prepare our troop for our presentation before Tsar Nicholas and his Empress Alexsandra Feodorovna.

There were eleven men in our group, plus me. We were drawn from the wider area around Moskva, but bragging aside, Vladimir and I were the stars of the show.

We had a joint act, with a quadrangle, jumping and shashka work, but our own little act was the best one. It began with Vladimir and I standing in Sarda's saddle, with me just behind him, one hand in the air, waving at the audience. We would then do a lift, ending up with my standing upon Vladimir's shoulders—at a full gallop.

It was a truly tricky maneuver, and one that few ever attempted. We lived, ate and breathed *džigitovka*. In any spare time, we worked out together— running, press-ups, sit-ups— we needed all the strength we could muster, and on the day of the performance for the Tsar Nicholas and Tsarina Alexandra Feodorovna, we triumphed.

During our bows to their Excellencies, the Empress Alexandra Feodorovna beckoned us closer.

"Your skills," she said, "for such young people are to be rewarded. I should like to see you both again." She paused for a moment. "Perhaps," she glanced at the tsar, who lifted an eyebrow at her, and then turned back to us, "you would like to attend the ball at the Kremlin tomorrow night?"

I swallowed hard.

"We should be honored, your Excellencies," Vladimir said, his voice smooth.

"We will see you there." The tsarina nodded and turned back toward her husband, dismissing us.

I curtsied as gracefully as I could, holding a pair of reins and wearing jodhpurs and boots, lacking the essential skirts. Vladimir drew me to my feet and escorted me away.

"A ball at the Kremlin?" I blinked and took a deep breath. "However will I find a ball dress before tomorrow night?"

"You have none?" He looked at me, jaw dropped.

I peered from beneath my brows. "How many balls have I attended since we met?"

He stared at me. "Well…"

"Exactly. I attended the end of year cadets ball with you last year, but that dress will hardly be suitable for an audience," I indicated my breeches and boots, "other than this, of course, with the tsar and tsarina. It's easy for you. You simply need your Training School dress uniform."

"Sisters. Yes, that's it." He spun to face me. "Olga and Sonja will have a dress to fit you."

My jaw dropped. His sisters were elegant young ladies. I'd been introduced to them before, but they hadn't seemed impressed by the stable girl performing with their brother. "But they live a full day's ride away. I'd never be able to ride there and return and still take care of my stable duties."

"I'll go. I can get one of the other lads to do my work for me, if your father permits."

"I permit," he said, walking up in time to hear the end of the conversation.

"Thank you, sir. I have three sisters, most of them close in size to Tatiana. With your permission, I will leave as soon as I cool out my horse."

"We'll take care of that and inform the headmaster. Well done, both of you. Your performance was without equal," he said, taking the reins of Vladimir's horse and leading him back toward the barn.

"Papa," I said, and he turned. I reached out for Sarda's reins. "Thank you, for all you've done for me, for us." I glanced at Vladimir's retreating back.

He handed them to me and hugged me, his eyes glistening with unshed tears. "You have made me so proud, both you and Vladimir. What a team you make."

"We could've never done it without you."

"Soon he will be finished here and must enter the tsar's army." He took back Sarda's reins and together we began walking the sweating horses. "Have you considered what you will do then?" His eyes looked at me—through me— and I shuddered, then swallowed and looked at the floor.

"I honestly do not know, Papa."

"A life of horses is hard for a man, much less a woman, and I won't be around forever."

My eyes snapped up to his. "What?" For the first time, I saw his weathered visage, the grayness of his skin at the edges, and my stomach clenched. "Papa, are you ill?"

He took a deep breath. "I'm not sure, but my heart, it does funny things sometimes. Not badly, but it's enough to give me pause—to question and to ensure you are provided for."

The walls of the Kremlin swayed around me. Papa was my rock, although I'd been increasingly leaning on Vladimir as we had become close friends, and now, it seems, something more.

"Have you been to a doctor, Papa?" Knowing her hadn't.

"No, but there is little they could do."

"You don't know that…"

"Trust me, I know. Anyway, *princessa*, you will be going to the ball and dancing the night away on the arm of your prince.

"Will you becoming?"

"The invitation was only for the two of you, but I will be awaiting your return with bated breath." I offered the horse a few sips of water from a bucket then pulled Sarda away and we resumed our walk.

"This will be my first ball without you, Papa…" I searched his face, seeking to know the extent of his sickness, but nothing showed.

"My *solnishko* has grown up." New tears in his eyes threatened to fall. "You will be the loveliest woman there."

Woman.

I'd never thought of myself as that…it would take some time to sink in.

Due out soon! Look for it!

Sign up for Lizzi's VIP Reader Club to hear about new releases and specials, plus get your free sampler gift at www.lizzitremayne/VIPGREEN

*Thank you for reading.
I hope you enjoyed Greener Pastures Calling.*

*Join Lizzi's VIP Reader Club to hear about new release
and specials, plus get your free book!*

It's right here:

www.lizzitremayne/VIPGREEN

www.ingramcontent.com/pod-product-compliance
Lightning Source LLC
Chambersburg PA
CBHW051651040426
42446CB00009B/1082